Atlas of
Vascular Surgery

Atlas of Vascular Surgery

Second Edition

Christopher K. Zarins, M.D.

Chidester Professor of Surgery
Stanford University
Chief of Vascular Surgery
Stanford University Medical Center
Stanford, California

Bruce L. Gewertz, M.D.

Dallas B. Phemister Professor
Chairman, Department of Surgery
The University of Chicago Pritzker School of Medicine
Chief, Section of Vascular Surgery
The University of Chicago Medical Center
Chicago, Illinois

Illustrated by Kathy Hirsh

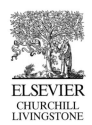

ELSEVIER
CHURCHILL
LIVINGSTONE

ELSEVIER
CHURCHILL
LIVINGSTONE

The Curtis Center
170 S Independence Mall W 300E
Philadelphia, PA 19106

ATLAS OF VASCULAR SURGERY, SECOND EDITION   ISBN 0-443-06592-6

Previous edition copyrighted 1989

International Standard Book Number 0-443-06592-6

Publishing Director: Anne Lenehan

Printed in the United States of America

Last digit is the print number: 9   8   7   6   5   4   3   2   1

Dedication

*This book is dedicated to our patients whose bravery
in the face of illness continues to inspire us
and
to our wives, Zinta and Diane, who have provided unfailing support
for our professional efforts with great personal sacrifice.*

Preface

Since the first edition of this vascular atlas in 1993, vascular surgery has continued to grow and evolve as a specialty devoted to the care of patients with vascular disease. Aided by improvements in diagnostic imaging, perioperative care, endovascular strategies and open surgical techniques, today's vascular specialists continue to treat some of the most difficult problems in medicine while achieving outcomes that our talented predecessors would envy. In most centers, vascular surgeons now provide the entire spectrum of invasive and noninvasive diagnostic studies and have the skills to apply both operative and endovascular therapies as needed. Important insights gained from this continuity of care have lowered the morbidity of atherosclerotic disease and furthered the basic and translational research which will allow us to provide even better patient care in the future.

The current edition of the ***Atlas of Vascular Surgery*** has been extensively modified to reflect today's practice of vascular surgery. An entirely new section on the endovascular treatment of aortic aneurysms has been added. Procedures have been updated to incorporate new operative approaches and adjunctive techniques. Additional information on the natural history, diagnostic evaluation, and indications for treatment has been provided to introduce each main section of the text.

Aided by the superb illustrative talents of our long-time collaborator Kathy Hirsch, we have attempted to communicate both the sequence and nuance of a wide range of arterial procedures. We focus on the judgments and techniques that we personally employ in our day-to-day practices at Stanford University and the University of Chicago and make no claim that these are the only successful approaches to these clinical challenges. That said, it is our hope that this latest edition continues to function as a concise and helpful resource for practicing surgeons who, like us, are privileged to care for patients with these challenging vascular problems.

Christopher K. Zarins, M.D.
Bruce L. Gewertz, M.D.

Contents

SECTION I

Aortic Arch and Extracranial Cerebrovascular Procedures

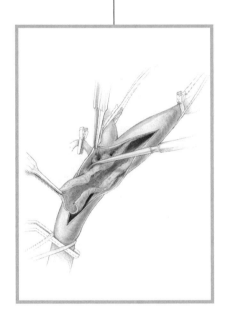

Patients with atherosclerotic or other obstructive lesions of the aortic arch and extracranial vessels may present with symptoms of embolization or flow limitation. Others may be asymptomatic, yet harbor lesions threatening sudden occlusion or other untoward symptoms. As noninvasive diagnostic methods including duplex carotid imaging and magnetic resonance (MR) and computed tomography (CT) angiograms have become more widely used, a greater percentage of patients are diagnosed before the onset of symptoms. In these patients, preemptive surgical procedures can only be justified if the mortality and morbidity of the intervention is low and if the benefit to the patient is clear. This section includes a wide range of surgical procedures addressing cerebrovascular disease in its broadest sense. The specific indications for each procedure are discussed, and outcomes and complications relating to each procedure are presented.

In this text we do not specifically address carotid angioplasty and stenting. Such procedures undoubtedly are useful in managing some patients with extracranial and intracranial disease. While the specific indications and long-term outcomes await better definition, we now apply these procedures in patients with relative contraindications to surgery, such as neck irridation, multiple previous procedures, and high preoperative cardiac risk.

Irrespective of the specific artery involved, any consideration of surgical intervention to decrease cerebrovascular risk mandates a thorough evaluation of cardiac status. This would include, at a minimum, taking a careful history centering on symptoms of coronary artery disease or congestive heart failure, as well as a broad discussion of risk factors including smoking history, hyperlipidemia, diabetes mellitus, hypertension, and obesity. A thorough neurologic history also is critical in such patients. Patients should be queried as to whether they have experienced headaches or changes in vision, including monocular blindness, partial or total field defects, and other visual disturbances. The occurrence of "migraine headaches" should be documented together with any subtle changes in cognition, stamina, or speech. The patient's perception of extremity weakness and sensory deficits should be explored, and any disquieting sensations including vertigo, syncope, or lightheadedness should be documented.

Physical examination should include a thorough vascular examination with particular attention to auscultation of the infraclavicular, supraclavicular, and cervical regions. Blood pressure measurements should be performed on both upper extremities to document any differences that may imply brachiocephalic disease. Attention should be paid to the rate and rhythm of the heartbeat. A careful and complete neurologic examination must be carried out to include specific evaluations of cranial nerves and objective testing of mentation, coordination, and other cognitive functions as indicated.

The thoroughness of the cardiac evaluation depends on the magnitude of the procedure and the patient's personal history. A minimum evaluation includes an electrocardiogram on all patients. The next level of inquiry may include an echocardiogram both at rest and during stress, as well as thallium perfusion studies with and without exertion or pharmacologic challenge. Occasionally, a patient may require a preoperative coronary angiogram to fully evaluate the coronary anatomy.

Depending on the specific indication, anatomy, and planned procedure, patients may require CT or MR imaging. Individual decisions need to be made as to whether noninvasive imaging using duplex ultrasound or MR angiography is satisfactory or selective arteriograms with intraarterial injections of contrast are required.

Carotid Artery Surgery

Carotid endarterectomy has become one of the most commonly performed vascular operations. To achieve combined morbidity and mortality rates of less than 5% with permanent neurologic deficit rates of less than 2%, attention must be paid to anesthetic management and to the technical aspects of the surgery. In addition, appropriate patient selection and thorough preoperative evaluation is essential. With such care and planning, a wide variety of anesthetic agents and intraoperative monitoring techniques achieve comparable results. It appears that the single most important factor in minimizing neurologic complications is technical precision in performing the endarterectomy.

We prefer general endotracheal anesthesia with intraoperative electroencephalographic monitoring to detect cerebral ischemia. An intraluminal shunt can be used "routinely" or "selectively" if cerebral ischemic changes are detected by electroencephalography (approximately 30% of patients).

Specific Indications

Symptomatic patients with severe atherosclerotic lesions of the carotid bifurcation commonly present with repeated symptoms of embolization either to the middle cerebral artery distribution or the retinal artery and its branches (amaurosis fugax). Prospective randomized studies have shown that most patients with carotid bifurcation lesions greater than 50% of diameter who present with symptoms should be considered for intervention or surgery. That said, it is occasionally difficult to define the specific source of embolization in patients with diffuse disease and multiple lesions. It is particularly important to exclude the innominate artery on the right or the origin of the left carotid artery from the aortic arch as a source of atherosclerotic debris.

The duplex scan can often provide information that allows the surgeon to pinpoint the most likely source of the emboli. These ultrasound imaging and velocity measurements can often indicate innominate artery or common carotid disease by direct visualization or by low blood flow velocities proximal to the carotid bifurcation. Distal (intracranial) stenoses are suggested by low or reduced diastolic flow in the distal internal carotid artery past the bifurcation lesion.

Irrespective of the clarity of these measures, if a patient presents with suggestions of brachiocephalic or intracranial disease and/or atypical symptoms, MR or selective angiography may be required. In our practice, this is necessary in approximately 20% of patients. Such atypical symptoms could include vertebrobasilar insufficiency, unusual visual field defects, and symptoms that could be more properly explained by contralateral ischemia or embolization. Classic "lateralizing" symptoms that might obviate the need for angiography include cortical symptoms ipsilateral to the lesion (such as expressive aphasia, particularly common in left carotid lesions), contralateral monoparesis or hemiparesis, and unilateral intermittent monocular blindness. As noted earlier, it is particularly important to exclude cardiac sources for emboli. Evaluation should include electrocardiogram or Holter monitoring if arrhythmia is suspected, as well as echocardiography to exclude valvular lesions such as aortic valve disease, mitral valve disease or prolapse, and atrial or ventricular thrombus.

Consideration of intervention in an asymptomatic patient with carotid atheroma is often a difficult decision. In practice, we rarely advocate surgery on asymptomatic lesions with less than a 70% diameter reduction even if associated with irregularity or ulceration. Because the projected neurologic risk of a 70% diameter lesion is approximately 3% to 5% per year, the decision to proceed with carotid endarterectomy mandates that the patient's overall perioperative risk is relatively low and that an individual's projected life span will afford some reasonable benefit in quality of life and long-term reduction in stroke risk. That said, age per se is not a contraindication to surgery for either symptomatic or asymptomatic patients. It is occasionally useful to obtain an infused CT scan or MR image of asymptomatic patients to determine whether previous, but unrecognized, cortical infarcts have occurred. In some series, as many as 20% of patients will manifest such "silent" infarcts. The demonstration of previous small infarcts may tip the balance toward a more active approach to carotid endarterectomy.

Complications

The most devastating nonfatal complication of carotid endarterectomy is perioperative stroke. Causes of stroke include embolization during dissection of the carotid or following restoration of flow, thrombosis of the endarterectomy site with or without embolization, and, finally, cerebral ischemia during intraoperative occlusion. Neurologic deficits may be evident immediately on awakening the patient or may occur in the postoperative period. Rarely, patients may present 3 to 7 days later with cerebral edema (reperfusion edema).

In the event that a patient awakens in the operating room with a neurologic deficit, it is usually prudent to reanesthetize the patient and immediately reexpose the carotid artery. At that time, the patency of the endarterectomy is determined with a handheld Doppler probe. In the event that the carotid endarterectomy site is occluded, heparinization and repeat arteriotomy can be carried out and the cause of thrombosis determined.

If the carotid arteries were still patent by Doppler examination, we would favor an intraoperative angiogram with intracranial views to attempt to determine the cause of the stroke, the adequacy of the endarterectomy and the arterial closure, and options for remediation. Any defect at the site of endarterectomy of closure must be repaired. If a distal embolus is recognized, the nature of the embolus would determine what options were available for treatment. For example, if no thrombus is noted near the endarterectomy site and a filling defect is observed in the distal middle cerebral artery or its branches, it could be concluded that the embolization reflected atherosclerotic debris. Alternatively, if thrombus is identified in the endarterectomy site, distal embolic material might well be dislodged thrombus and localized short-term fibrinolytic therapy might be considered. If direct visualization of the endarterectomy reveals no technical errors but rather a thrombogenic surface leading to platelet deposition, replacement of the carotid bifurcation may be required. Options would include polytetrafluoroethylene graft or autogenous saphenous vein.

If a patient awakens neurologically intact and then experiences a neurologic deficit in the first few hours after surgery, the most immediate decision is whether to return the patient to the operating room for urgent evaluation or to treat in a supportive fashion. In the rare instance that this occurs, an expeditious duplex scan should be carried out to determine the patency of the carotid and the status of the carotid bifurcation. Treatment decisions should be based on these objective data, as well as the patient's condition and progression. In general, if no defects are demonstrated at the site of the endarterectomy and the patient is improving, supportive therapy with anticoagulation and careful observation may be appropriate. In contrast, if any defect whatsoever is noted at the bifurcation or the patient's condition is not resolving, it is always safer to return the patient to the operating room for reexploration and possible revision as detailed above.

Temporary or permanent injury to cranial nerves is another significant complication of carotid endarterectomy. The most commonly injured nerves include the superior laryngeal nerve, vagus nerve, hypoglossal nerve, and marginal mandibular branch of the facial nerve. The incidence rate of such cranial nerve injuries is variable, with temporary deficits evident in 3% to 10% of patients and permanent deficits evident in 1% to 2% of patients. Avoidance of such complications requires careful operative dissection and specifically minimization of any traction on the underside of the mandible that leads to marginal mandibular nerve dysfunction. In general, reoperation is not indicated even if cranial nerve injury is diagnosed in the postoperative period.

Wound hematomas occasionally will occur especially in patients treated with antiplatelet agents perioperatively. To minimize the incidence of this complication, our practice has included the placement of small suction drains for the first 24 hours. We also use protamine to reverse heparinization before wound closure. The dreaded secondary complication of neck hematomas is airway obstruction. If any respiratory compromise is noted, the patient must be immediately returned to the operating room for evacuation of the hematoma and appropriate hemostasis.

A   The patient is placed supine on the operating table with a shoulder roll. The neck is extended and the head is rotated 45 degrees to the opposite side. Electrodes are placed on the scalp for continuous electroencephalographic monitoring if "selective" shunting is practiced. An incision is made that extends along the anterior border of the sternocleidomastoid muscle over the carotid artery. This provides excellent exposure, a good cosmetic result, and permits extension superiorly and inferiorly if required during the course of the operation. Transverse incisions in the skin folds of the neck can be made, but in our experience they do not provide as good exposure of the distal internal carotid artery.

B   Insert demonstrates the relationship between carotid artery branches and cranial nerves. Note the branch of external carotid artery to sternocleidomastoid muscle, which occasionally tethers hypoglossal nerve.

C   The platysma muscle is divided and the anterior border of the sternocleidomastoid (SCM) muscle is identified. Sharp dissection is carried along the anterior border of the SCM to identify the underlying internal jugular vein. The facial vein is identified as it crosses over the carotid bifurcation. The vein is suture ligated and divided to expose the underlying carotid artery. The omohyoid muscle may be divided, if necessary, for better exposure of the common carotid artery. The carotid sheath is opened and the common carotid artery is carefully encircled proximal to the bifurcation.

     Control of the superior thyroid artery is obtained, avoiding injury to the superior laryngeal nerve that often crosses over the first portion of the artery. A silastic tape is placed around the external carotid artery. The tissue between the external and internal carotid artery is then infiltrated with 1% xylocaine to anesthetize the carotid sinus nerve. The hypoglossal nerve, which crosses the external and internal carotid arteries superior to the bifurcation, is identified and protected from injury. The ansa hypoglossi (ansa cervicalis) may be seen exiting from the hypoglossal nerve. It is rarely necessary to divide the ansa cervicalis, but this can be performed for adequate exposure of the internal carotid artery, if necessary. Dissection of the distal internal carotid is then carried out and a silastic tape is passed around the artery for control. It is sometimes helpful to divide the muscular branch of the external carotid artery that crosses the hypoglossal nerve to mobilize the nerve medially, thereby improving exposure of the distal internal carotid artery. If the plaque extends well beyond the bifurcation, division of the digastric muscle allows exposure of the distal internal carotid artery to the level of the styloid process. To avoid embolization, the carotid bifurcation itself should not be dissected at this time.

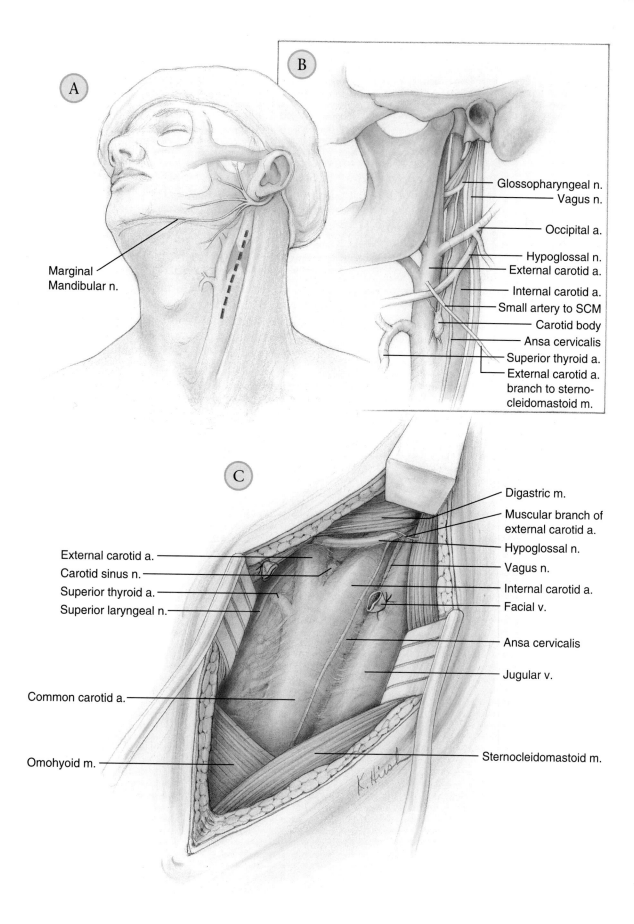

A

Marginal
Mandibular n.

B

Glossopharyngeal n.
Vagus n.
Occipital a.
Hypoglossal n.
External carotid a.
Internal carotid a.
Small artery to SCM
Carotid body
Ansa cervicalis
Superior thyroid a.
External carotid a.
branch to sterno-
cleidomastoid m.

C

Digastric m.
Muscular branch of
external carotid a.
Hypoglossal n.
Vagus n.
Internal carotid a.
Facial v.
Ansa cervicalis
Jugular v.
Sternocleidomastoid m.

External carotid a.
Carotid sinus n.
Superior thyroid a.
Superior laryngeal n.

Common carotid a.

Omohyoid m.

K. Hisal

D   After control of the common, external, and internal carotid arteries is obtained, the surgeon should verify with the anesthesiologist that the patient is hemodynamically stable. Blood pressure should be maintained at normal levels during the period of carotid occlusion. The patient is systemically heparinized, and if continuous electroencephalographic monitoring is being carried out, the character of the tracings are ascertained. Clamps are then applied to the distal internal carotid artery, external carotid artery, superior thyroid artery, and common carotid artery. We use Heifetz vascular clips for the distal branches because they are relatively atraumatic and do not obstruct the operative field. Dissection and mobilization of the carotid bifurcation should be completed only after the common carotid artery is clamped.

E   An arteriotomy is made in the common carotid artery and extended along the lateral wall of the carotid bifurcation into the internal carotid artery. The arteriotomy is terminated just past the plaque in the internal carotid. In some instances with very extensive calcific lesions, it may be impossible to locate the pinpoint lumen within the plaque. One should simply extend the incision along the plaque and reenter the lumen superiorly distal to the stenosis. The distal internal carotid artery clamp is momentarily released to confirm the presence of back bleeding from the distal circulation. If electroencephalographic abnormalities develop at any time, an intraluminal shunt should be placed (see Fig. A, page 15).

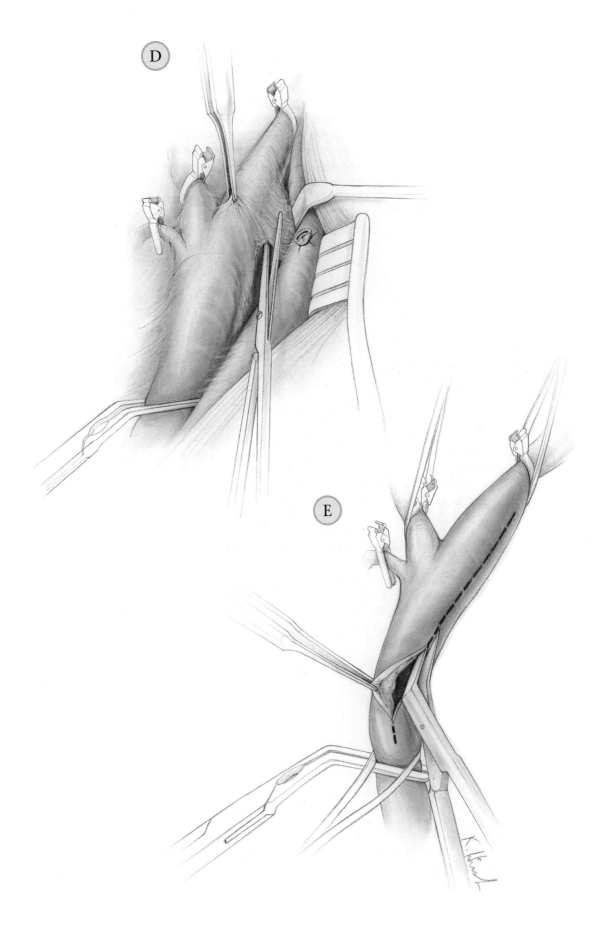

(F) Heparinized saline is used to irrigate the lumen, and the lumen surface is carefully inspected. The presence of ulceration or intraluminal thrombus is noted. The endarterectomy is then performed using an endarterectomy spatula or elevator. It is most important to select the proper plane of endarterectomy in the outer portion of the media just below the external elastic lamina (EEL). The proper plane of dissection is most easily visualized in the thickest portion of the plaque. A circumferential layer of medial smooth muscle, adherent to the intimal plaque, should be removed with the specimen. Care must be exercised to avoid beginning different planes of dissection on the two sides of the arteriotomy. The plaque is sharply transected at the common carotid artery and an eversion endarterectomy is performed of the superior thyroid artery and external carotid artery. Finally, the distal end point of the plaque in the internal carotid is visualized and carefully disengaged from the underlying media.

(G) Demonstration of the layers of the artery wall with the proper plane of dissection in the outer portion of the media just below the EEL. The media in the thickest portion of the plaque is usually degenerated and is readily removed with the diseased intima. In the distal internal carotid artery, where the plaque becomes thin, the media is normal, and the plaque "feathers out" superficial to the internal elastic lamina (IEL). This natural transition and termination of plaque is usually distinct. If this area is not readily visible through the arteriotomy, the arteriotomy should be extended.

(H) The arteriotomy is irrigated with heparinized saline and carefully inspected under magnification. Residual shreds of circumferentially oriented medial smooth muscle cells are removed, and the distal internal carotid end point is carefully inspected. If the distal intima is not firmly adherent to the media, interrupted 7–0 tacking sutures are placed to avoid subintimal dissection and creation of a "flap valve." These tacking sutures should be oriented in a longitudinal direction to avoid constriction of the lumen. The transected plaque in the common carotid artery is carefully inspected. If significant residual plaque exists in the common carotid artery, the arteriotomy should be extended proximally and the plaque removed. Tacking sutures may also be necessary in the proximal common carotid artery. Even though the direction of blood flow usually will not result in subintimal dissection, oscillation of the intimal at this point can lead to resterosis. The external carotid orifice is carefully inspected and back bleeding is confirmed by releasing the clamp.

(I) Tacking sutures in the distal internal carotid artery should be placed in a longitudinal direction with one needle placed through the normal distal intima and the other through the endarterectomized surface. The knot should always be tied on the outside and should not be pulled too tightly to avoid puckering of the vessel or tearing of the suture through the thin intima.

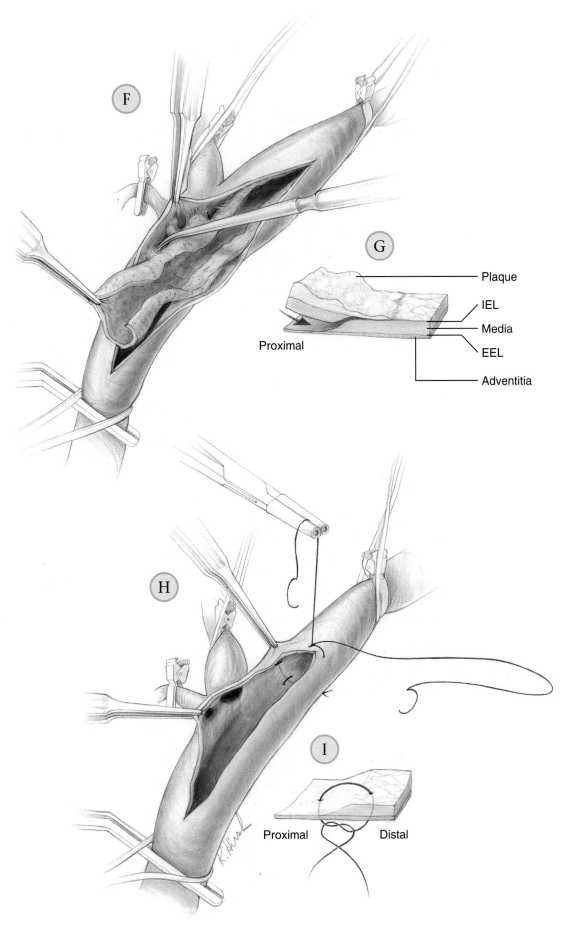

Plaque

IEL

Media

EEL

Adventitia

Proximal

Proximal   Distal

The arteriotomy can occasionally be closed primarily with a continuous 6–0 monofilament nonabsorbable suture. The sutures are begun from the ends of the arteriotomy. Precise closure with closely placed sutures is essential; great care must be taken to avoid stenosis. If the arteriotomy must be extended past the carotid bulb into a small distal internal carotid artery, a patch may be required to avoid lumen stenosis.

In our most recent series, we patch approximately 50% of carotid endarterectomies using a specially tailored woven Dacron or polytetrafluoroethylene patch. Common indications for patching include: (1) a small internal carotid artery less than 2.5 mm; (2) history or expectation of continued smoking; (3) history of recurrent stenoses in cerebrovascular or other vascular beds; and (4) female sex. The patch must be appropriately sized to avoid creating too large of a carotid bifurcation that may result in stasis and potential thrombus formation.

The suture line is briefly paused nearing completion to allow appropriate flushing of distal and proximal arteries. The arteriotomy is then carefully filled with heparinized saline to allow evacuation of all residual air and other debris. The suture line is then completed. Flow is restored first through the external carotid artery and, after three to five heartbeats, the internal carotid artery clamp is removed. This minimizes the risk for any residual air or particles entering the cerebral circulation.

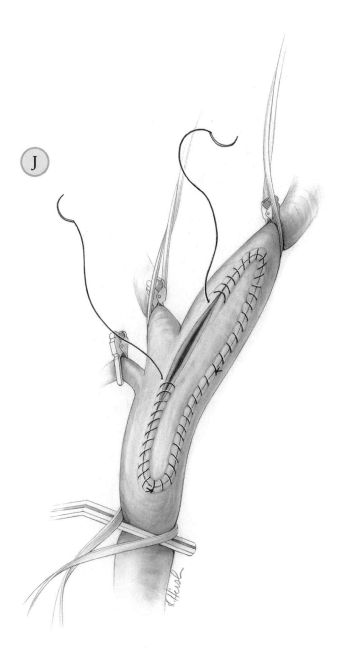

In most patients, collateral circulation will maintain adequate cerebral blood flow during the period of carotid occlusion. However, in 10% to 20% of patients, significant intraoperative ischemia develops. This ischemia can be prevented by placing an intraluminal shunt between the common carotid and distal internal carotid artery Some surgeons elect to use a shunt in all cases of carotid endarterectomy even though only a minority of patients require shunts. Because shunts occasionally interfere with visualization of the distal portion of the endarterectomy, we shunt "selectively." We use continuous intraoperative electroencephalographic monitoring and shunt only those patients who demonstrate intraoperative ischemia or present with clinical criteria indicating increased risk for perioperative neurologic deficits. These include: (1) recent stroke or reversible ischemic neurologic deficit; (2) contralateral internal carotid occlusion or critical stenosis; and (3) significant intracranial disease, carotid siphon stenosis, or an incomplete circle of Willis.

Exposure and preparation for carotid endarterectomy is carried out as described on pages 7–9. The patient is heparinized. The arteriotomy is begun in the common carotid artery and extended through the carotid bulb to the distal internal carotid artery past the plaque. The internal carotid artery Heifetz clip is removed, and back bleeding is allowed to occur through the distal internal carotid artery. A balloon-tipped intraluminal carotid shunt is carefully advanced into the lumen of the internal carotid artery. Blood flow retrograde through the shunt confirms proper positioning and evacuates air from the lumen of the shunt. The proximal end is then guided into the common carotid artery and the balloon is inflated for hemostasis. A Dacron umbilical tape is wrapped around the common carotid artery to slightly constrict the common carotid artery and to prevent the force of blood from pushing the balloon out during the course of the endarterectomy. Care must be exercised in placing the catheter so that atherosclerotic debris, air bubbles, and blood clots do not enter the system. This is best accomplished by making a generous arteriotomy so that the artery lumen can be clearly visualized. Care must be exercised not to overinflate the distal balloon and rupture the internal carotid artery. In cases where the distal internal carotid artery is small, it is not necessary to inflate the distal balloon. When the shunt is in place, the stopcock on the side arm is turned to demonstrate that blood is indeed flowing in the shunt. Overinflation of either balloon can angulate or obstruct the tip of the shunt and prevent blood flow even though the shunt is in proper position. Should electroencephalographic abnormalities persist or recur after shunt placement, shunt flow must be reexamined to rule out the possibility of kinking of the plastic tubing or other mechanical malfunction.

After the shunt is secured and demonstrated to be functional, the endarterectomy is carried out as described on page 11.

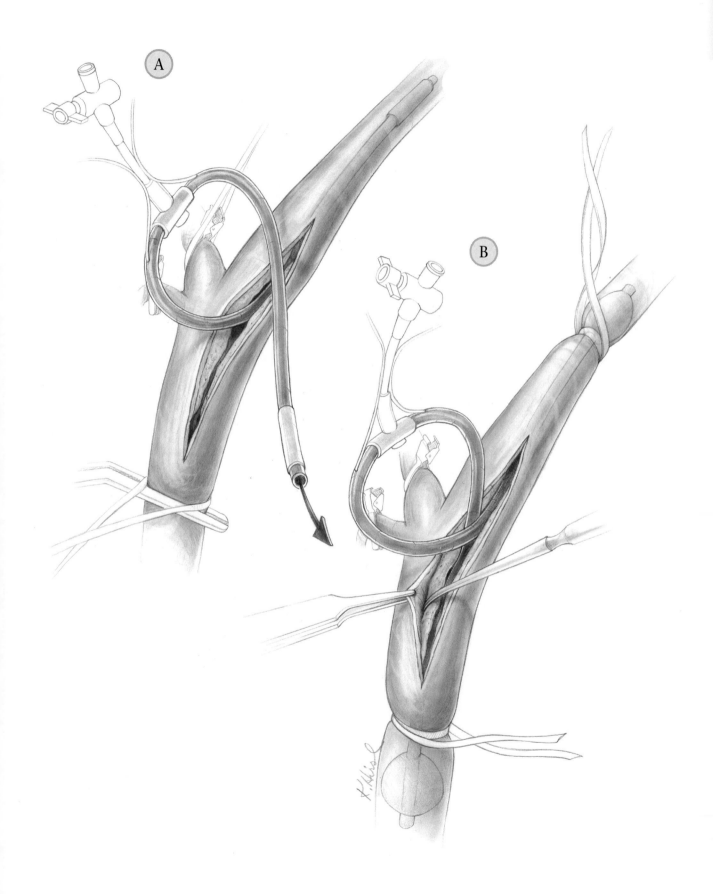

The arteriotomy is closed with the shunt still in place. When sutures can no longer be placed easily, the distal balloon is deflated and the internal carotid portion of the shunt is clamped and removed. A Heifetz clip is placed on the distal internal carotid artery. The proximal lumen is then deflated, and the shunt is completely removed. The proximal carotid artery is flushed, and a clamp is applied. Arteriotomy closure can then be completed. The external carotid clamps are removed, and the initial blood flow from the common carotid artery is allowed to proceed out the external carotid artery. After several seconds, the internal carotid artery is unclamped.

In instances where a patient does not tolerate even brief periods of carotid occlusion, reclamping of the common carotid artery after removal of the shunt can be avoided by using a small vascular clamp to control the arteriotomy after shunt removal. This allows immediate revascularization of the internal carotid artery while the arteriotomy is carefully closed.

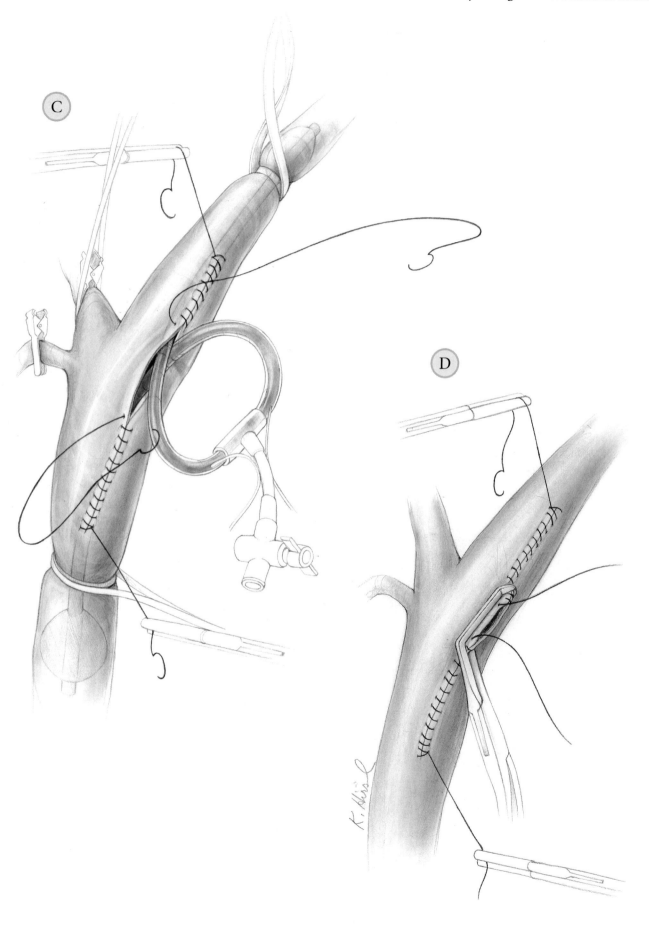

On rare instances, complications may be encountered when using balloon shunts. Overzealous inflation of the distal balloon, especially with saline, in very small internal carotid arteries can result in intimal or transmural injury to the artery.

 Advancing the shunt more distally in the internal carotid artery with careful reinflation is necessary. Multiple small crossing branches of the internal jugular vein should be divided to afford more adequate distal exposure. The arteriotomy is then extended up and through the area of injury and a proper repair is carried out. Invariably, a patch is necessary to ensure an adequate closure without narrowing the internal carotid artery.

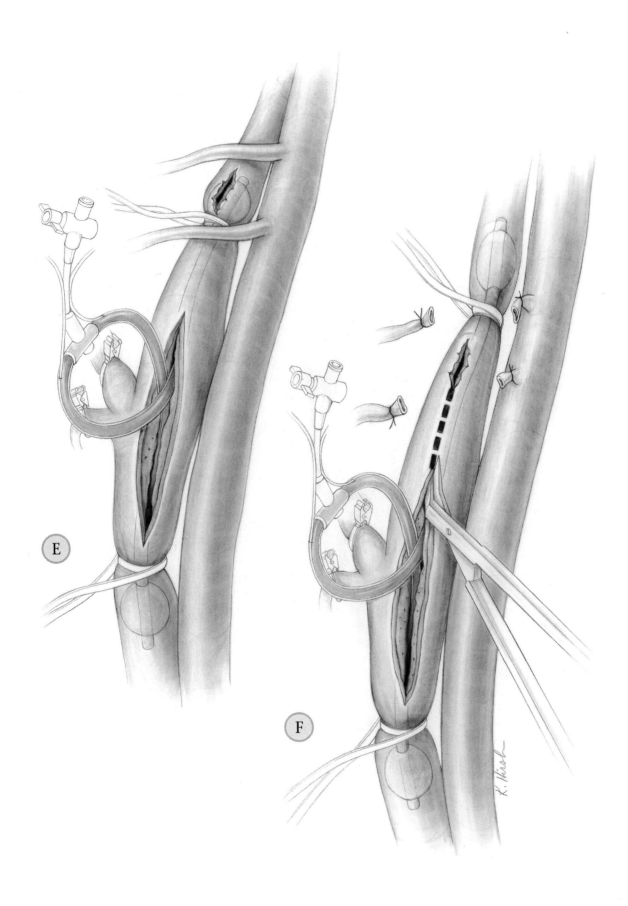

In situations where elongation and kinking of the carotid artery is symptomatic with or without significant atherosclerotic plaque at the carotid bifurcation, the internal carotid elongation should be corrected.

(A) After control and dissection of the carotid bifurcation, the origin of the proximal internal carotid artery is divided as it originates from the common carotid artery. The proximal incision is extended into the carotid biforcation. This facilitates endarterectomy of the plaque.

(B) The internal carotid artery is opened along its inner wall to the level necessary to straighten out the carotid kink.

(C) An eversion endarterectomy of the distal internal carotid artery is carried out. The distal end point should be visualized. If needed, an intraluminal shunt can be placed taking care to straighten the coil or kink before advancing the shunt.

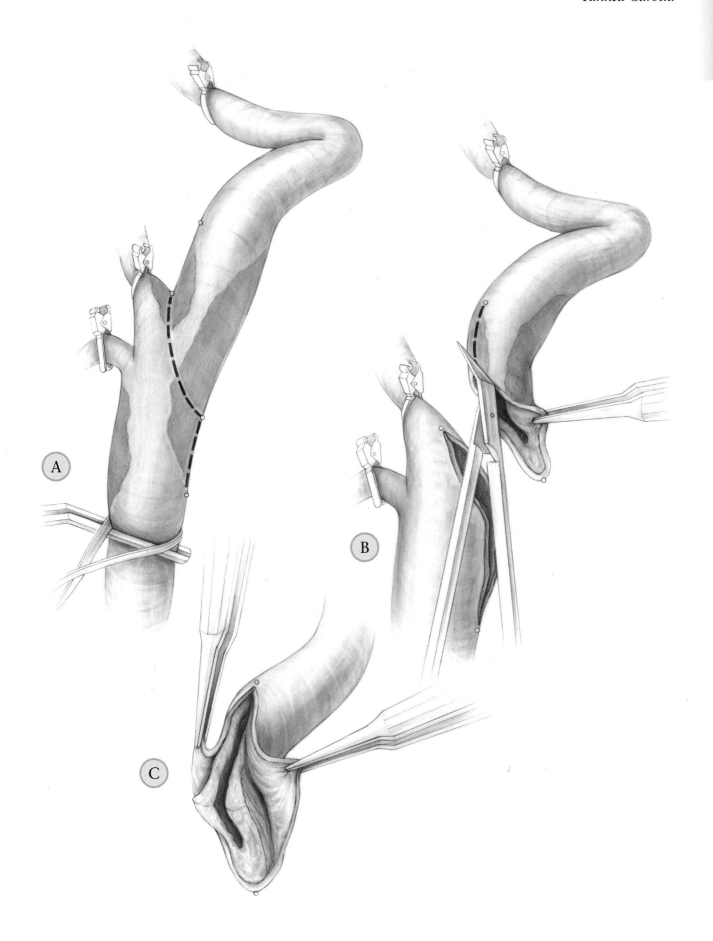

D Tacking sutures of interrupted 7–0 are used, if needed, to secure the distal end point, and the endarterectomized surface is carefully inspected.

E The spatulated internal carotid artery is then pulled down to straighten the kink. A primary anastomosis between the internal carotid artery and the common carotid artery is performed using continuous 6–0 monofilament suture. The back wall of the anastomosis is usually sewn from the inside of the artery. This provides the best visualization because rotation of the carotid may be cumbersome.

F Appropriate back flushing from the distal vessels is performed. The anastomosis is completed, and flow is restored to the external and then the internal carotid artery.

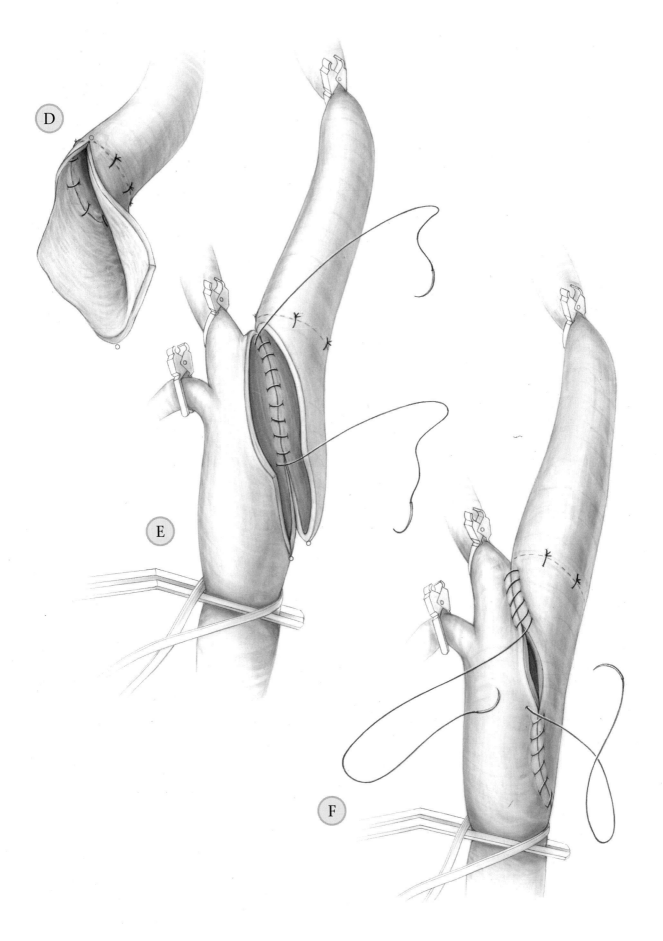

Elongation of the internal carotid artery can sometimes result in a 360-degree coil without significant carotid bifurcation stenosis. Such abnormalities are relatively rare, but can occasionally cause symptoms when the neck is rotated.

A   Demonstration of a coiled carotid.

B   After mobilization of the carotid and control proximally and distally, the coiled segment is resected.

C   A primary anastomosis of the internal carotid artery is performed in an end-to-end fashion.

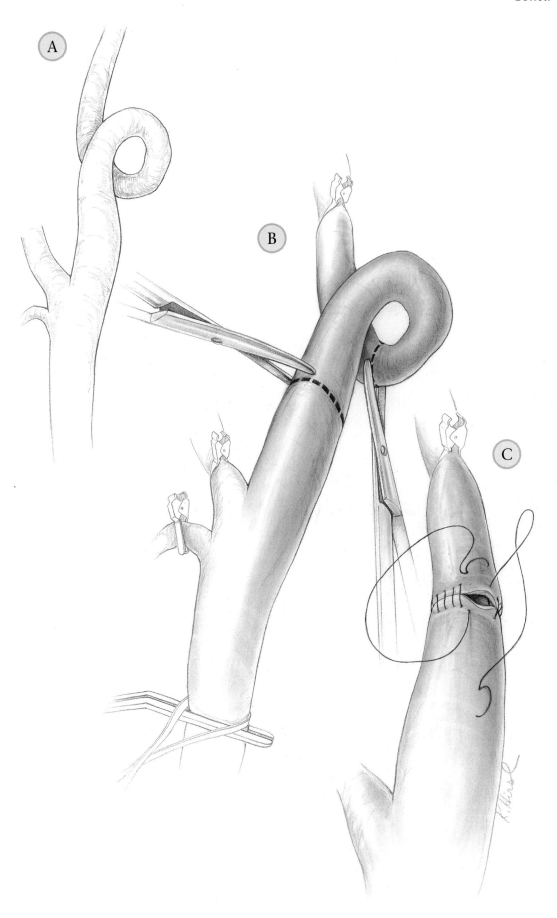

Approximately 5% to 10% of carotid endarterectomies are complicated by restenosis. Early restenosis (<2 years) is caused by either technical imperfection at the time of the initial surgery with residual atherosclerotic plaque or intimal flap or intimal hyperplasia. Recurrences after 2 years more frequently represent recurrent atherosclerotic disease. The incidence of atherosclerotic recurrences peaks more than 5 years after endarterectomy.

In most instances, intimal hyperplasia does not require operative repair unless the lesion is extremely stenotic (>80%) or is associated with emboli or other symptoms. In our experience, the smooth recurrent lesions caused by intimal hyperplasia are rarely associated with embolization. In contrast, atherosclerotic lesions occurring more than 5 years after endarterectomy have a natural history similar to the initial lesion and should be considered for operative intervention (see description on pages 7–13).

The morbidity of repeat carotid endarterectomy is generally increased over initial surgery. As a consequence, some surgeons favor carotid angioplasty and stenting in such situations. The principal complications of operative therapy include cranial nerve injury, because anatomic planes are obscured and identification and protection of nerves may be more difficult. Especially in patients who have undergone previous bilateral carotid endarterectomies, it is important to determine the status of their vocal cord movement and the function of other cranial nerves before the decision to move forward with a repeat endarterectomy. Irrespective of that status, utmost attention must be focused on preservation and avoidance of injury to cranial nerves.

(A) In recurrent lesions, we almost always obtain an angiogram to better delineate the distal and proximal extent of the lesion and to determine options for repair.

(B) Endarterectomy is rarely an option in early recurrence because the intimal hyperplastic lesion is not well suited to development of a subintimal dissection plane. Replacement is preferred. As shown here, after mobilization, the internal carotid is transected just proximal to the origin of the lesion, and a suitable distal point is selected.

(C) We prefer a small-diameter prosthetic graft, usually 5 or 6 mm. Polytetrafluoroethylene is the preferred interposition graft. Vein grafts are also useful, but they seem to offer little advantage in this particular position. The distal anastomosis is completed in an end-to-end fashion. The spatulated proximal anastomosis to the carotid bifurcation allows a wide diameter minimizing the chance of another recurrence.

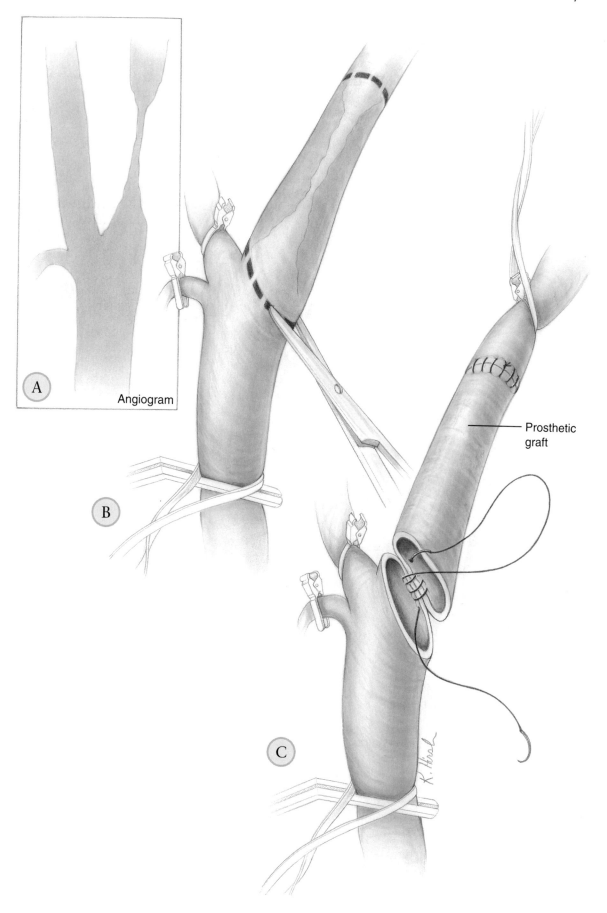

A

Angiogram

B

C

Prosthetic graft

An alternate technique for reconstruction of stenosed internal carotid arteries involves transposition of the external carotid to the internal carotid artery. Of course, this requires a patent and nondiseased external carotid of good caliber. As shown here, the same portion of internal carotid artery is resected, and the external carotid artery is divided.

 After ligation of the distal stump of the external carotid, the more proximal portion of the artery is rotated and anastomosed in an end-to-end fashion to the internal carotid above the lesion. It is important to close the stump of the excised internal carotid artery flush with the carotid bifurcation to avoid a stagnant area that could lead to thrombus deposition.

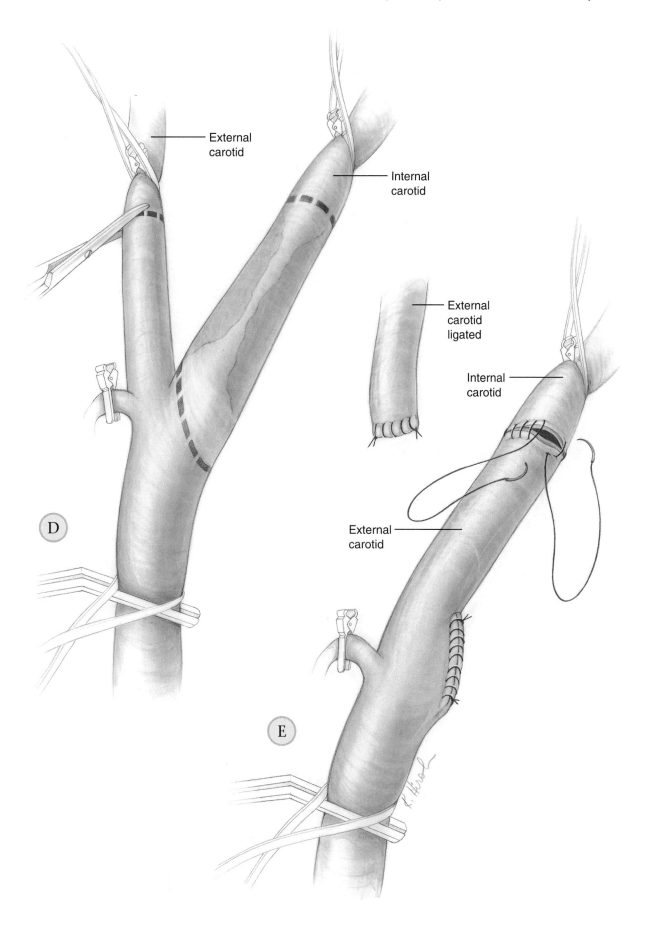

External
carotid

Internal
carotid

External
carotid
ligated

Internal
carotid

External
carotid

D

E

Fibromuscular dysplasia of the internal carotid artery can cause cerebrovascular symptoms due to focal stenoses or emboli. Although these lesions can be treated with balloon dilation, percutaneous dilation was not advisable in the past because distal embolization to the brain might occur. Therefore, we prefer intraoperative dilation that permits retrograde flushing of debris out the arteriotomy. It is possible that the continued development of "neuroprotective" intravascular devices may increase the utility of nonoperative angioplasties for these lesions.

The carotid bifurcation is gently dissected as described on pages 7–9. The superior thyroid and external carotid arteries are clamped. An arteriotomy is made in the carotid bulb proximal to the origin of the internal carotid artery.

Using balloon dilation under fluoroscopic control, the fibrotic bands in the distal internal carotid artery are dilated. Clamps are not applied to the distal internal carotid artery so that continued back bleeding from the distal internal carotid artery flushes debris out the arteriotomy. Alternatively, distal neuroprotective devices may be employed.

After completion of the dilation, the arteriotomy is closed with continuous 6–0 monofilament suture. Clamps are removed, and adequacy of the dilation is confirmed with intraoperative angiography.

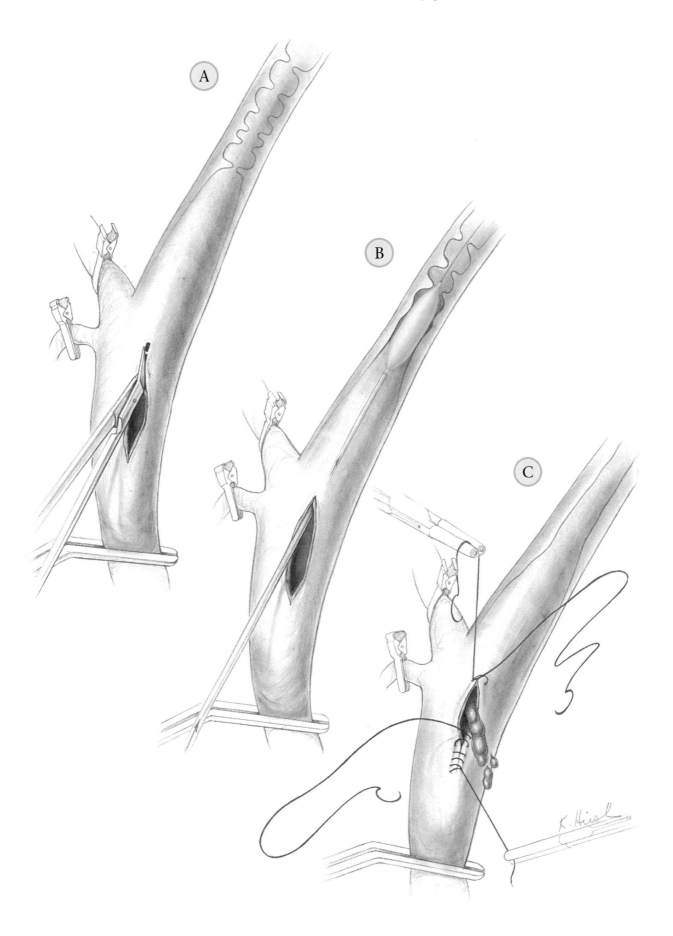

In patients with totally occluded common carotid and internal carotid arteries, the external carotid artery may function as an important source of collateral flow to the intracranial circulation. Hemispheric cerebrovascular symptoms may be relieved by revascularization of the external carotid artery. Xenon cerebral blood flow studies are useful in selecting patients for external carotid revascularization.

The patient is positioned supine on the operating table with a shoulder roll and extension of the neck. An incision is made along the anterior border of the sternocleidomastoid muscle for exposure of the carotid bifurcation (see description on page 7). A second incision is made transversely in the neck one fingerbreadth above the clavicle, the phrenic nerve is protected, and the anterior scalene muscle is divided to expose the subclavian artery distal to the vertebral artery. A suitable bypass graft is selected; this may be saphenous vein or 6 mm of polytetrafluoroethylene. The bypass is tunnelled underneath the sternocleidomastoid muscle. The proximal end-to-side anastomosis is made to the subclavian artery distal to the vertebral artery. A longitudinal arteriotomy is made in the external carotid artery. The graft is tailored in length to avoid kinking and anastomosed end-to-side to the external carotid artery.

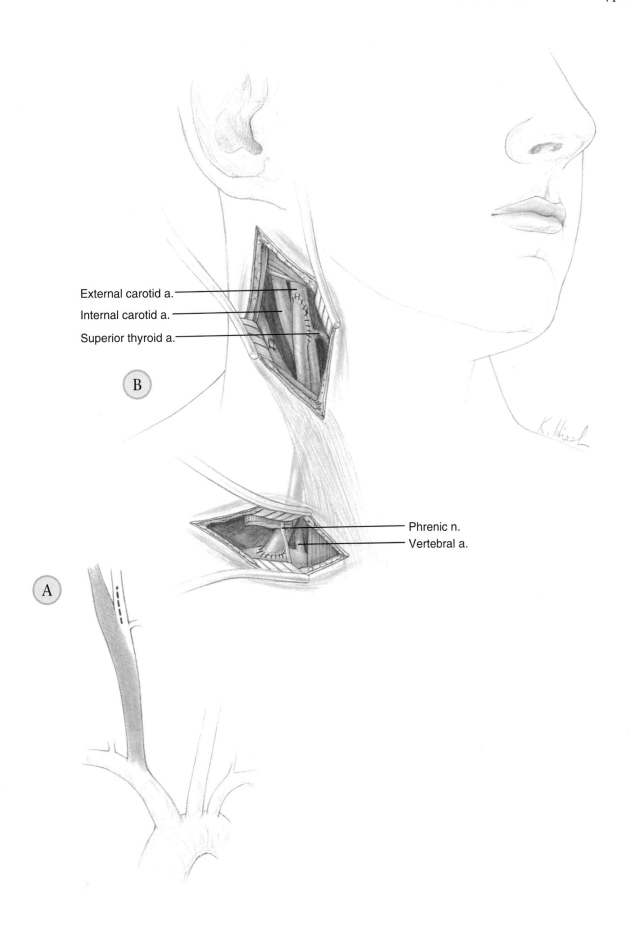

External carotid a.
Internal carotid a.
Superior thyroid a.

B

Phrenic n.
Vertebral a.

A

K. Hisl

Numerous communications exist between the intracranial circulation and the external carotid artery network. Under normal circumstances, the direction of flow in these communicating channels is from the internal carotid to the external carotid distribution. However, when the internal carotid artery is occluded, the direction of blood flow reverses and the external carotid artery becomes an important source of collateral flow to the brain.

A

Patients with internal carotid artery occlusion can be symptomatic from either stenosis of the proximal portion of the external carotid artery or embolization of thrombotic material from the cul-de-sac of the occluded internal carotid artery. Symptoms can include hemispheric transient ischemic attacks and amaurosis fugax. Cerebral blood flow measurements are useful in patient selection. Relief of a clinically significant external carotid artery stenosis in a patient with an internal carotid artery occlusion usually results in improvement in cerebral blood flow measurements.

B

Exposure and dissection of the carotid bifurcation is as described on pages 7–9. The proximal internal carotid artery is transected, and the arteriotomy is extended down the common carotid artery and into the external carotid artery.

C

An endarterectomy of the carotid bifurcation is performed with careful attention to the distal break point in the external carotid artery. The incision is extended further into the external carotid artery if necessary.

D

The arteriotomy is closed with a patch using continuous 6–0 monofilament suture. This procedure relieves the external carotid stenosis and eliminates the cul-de-sac of the occluded internal carotid artery.

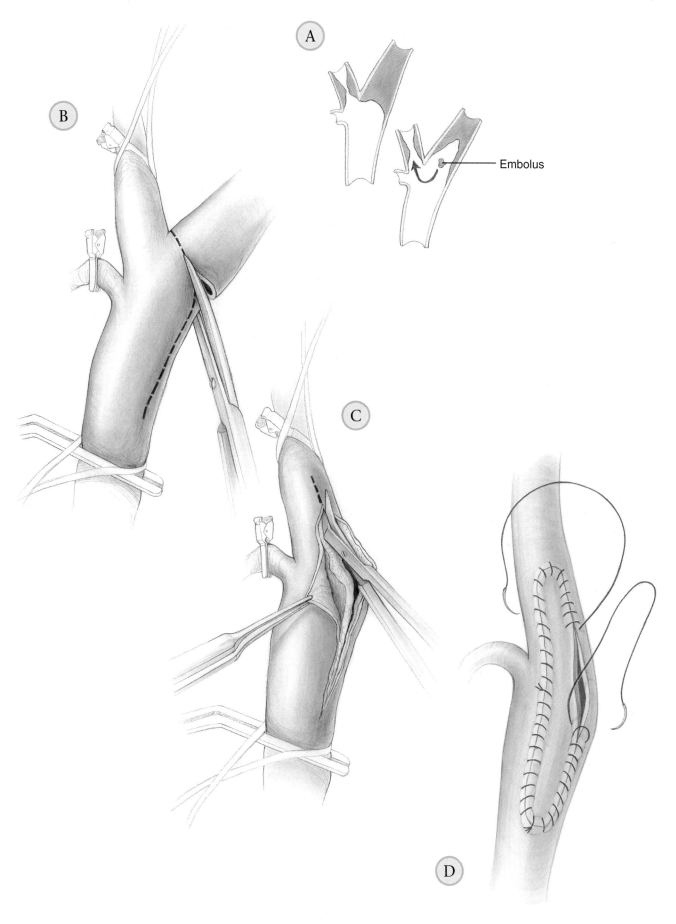

Embolus

9 • *External Carotid Endarterectomy with a Patch*

At times the bifurcation plaque extends far into the external carotid artery and cannot readily be removed by eversion endarterectomy during the standard carotid endarterectomy (see page 11). If poor back bleeding is obtained from the distal external carotid artery or a poor break point is obtained, the patency of the vessel should be determined. This may be assessed by intraoperative carotid imaging with duplex ultrasound, intraoperative angiography, or both. If obstruction of the external carotid artery is confirmed, repair is usually indicated.

 Reclamping of the common carotid artery is unnecessary and undesirable. A side biting vascular clamp can provide proximal vascular occlusion without obstructing flow to the internal carotid artery. A longitudinal arteriotomy is made in the external carotid artery, and endarterectomy of the residual atherosclerotic plaque is performed with direct visualization of the distal end point. Exposure of the external carotid artery more distally may be required.

 The external carotid endarterectomy is closed using a vein or prosthetic patch.

 The patch is tailored to an appropriate size and sutured in place.

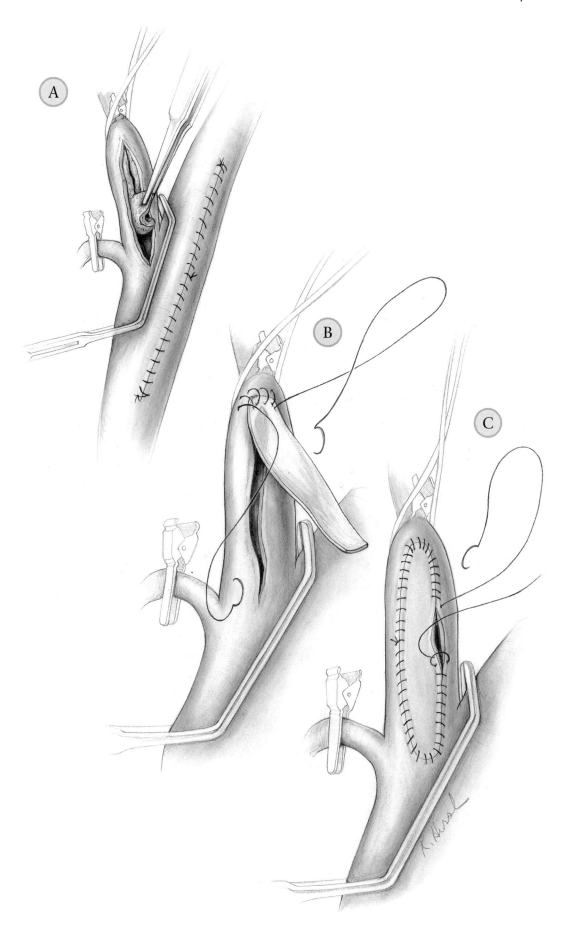

Operations for Vertebrobasilar Insufficiency

The most frequent symptoms of basilar insufficiency include nausea, vertigo, ipsilateral facial numbness, ipsilateral Horner's syndrome, and limb ataxia. Although ischemic symptoms are generally mild, true posterior fossa infarction can be progressive and lethal because of extensive edema and midbrain compression. While emboli can contribute to posterior cerebral and cerebellar ischemia, intermittent flow reductions in the vertebral or basilar arteries are the most common mechanism. Later, the thrombotic processes may involve the basilar artery proper or the basilar branch vessels that penetrate into the brainstem.

A classic syndrome of vertebrobasilar insufficiency ("subclavian steal syndrome") is associated with subclavian or innominate arterial occlusive disease. The subclavian origins of the vertebral arteries allow the vessels to function as collaterals for the upper extremity. The anatomic relation favors left-sided involvement by a ratio of approximately 4:1. During arm exercise, flow is "reversed" in the vertebral artery, and basilar arterial blood flow and perfusion pressure are decreased. Symptoms of posterior cerebral and cerebellar ischemia can result, especially if any flow-limiting carotid lesions are present. The diagnosis of subclavian steal syndrome is supported by patient reports of intermittent vertigo, lightheadedness, nausea, and vomiting intensified by arm exercise. Physical findings include supraclavicular bruits and 40 to 60 mm Hg blood pressure discrepancies between the arms. The differential diagnosis in patients of advanced age includes inner ear disorders and chronic subdural hematomas that may result from rather trivial trauma.

Symptomatic patients with multiple vertebral occlusive lesions or subclavian steal syndrome should be considered for elective surgery. Procedures described in this section include endarterectomy of the proximal vertebral artery or carotid–subclavian bypass to restore antegrade vertebral flow. In patients with severe stenoses or short-segment occlusions of the subclavian artery, angioplasty and stenting can also be considered. These less invasive approaches are best suited for infirm or high-risk patients with favorable anatomy.

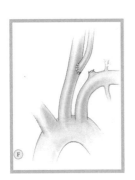

Revascularization of the subclavian artery can be accomplished by carotid–subclavian bypass or direct anastomosis of the subclavian artery to the common carotid artery. When the lesion is limited to the origin of the left subclavian artery and the subclavian artery lies close to the common carotid artery, the procedure of choice is a direct anastomosis between the side of the common carotid and transected subclavian artery (transposition). When the lesion is more extensive and extends to the origin of the vertebral artery, carotid–subclavian bypass is preferred.

The patient is positioned supine on the operating table with a shoulder roll beneath the shoulders. A transverse incision is made one fingerbreadth above the clavicle, and the platysma muscle is divided. The clavicular head of the sternocleidomastoid muscle is transected.

The internal jugular vein is identified just below the sternocleidomastoid muscle, mobilized, and retracted medially. Care must be taken to avoid injury to the thoracic duct. The descending cervical lymphatics join the thoracic duct at the junction of the subclavian vein and left internal jugular vein. The thoracic duct courses from posterior to anterior behind the jugular and subclavian veins to enter the superior border of the junction of these two veins. Should injury to the thoracic duct occur, the duct must be identified and ligated to avoid a lymph fistula. The internal jugular vein is gently retracted medially, and the underlying carotid artery is identified. The common carotid artery is dissected. The vagus nerve and stellate ganglion that lie behind the carotid artery must be protected from injury. The scalene fat pad is retracted laterally, and the anterior scalene muscle is identified lateral to the carotid artery. The phrenic nerve courses on the anterior surface of the scalene muscle and must be identified and preserved. The phrenic nerve is gently mobilized, and the anterior scalene muscle is transected. The muscle should be divided at an avascular area low in the neck near its origin from the first rib. Electrocautery should be avoided to prevent potential injury to the brachial plexus. After division of the scalene muscle, the underlying subclavian artery is visualized and dissected.

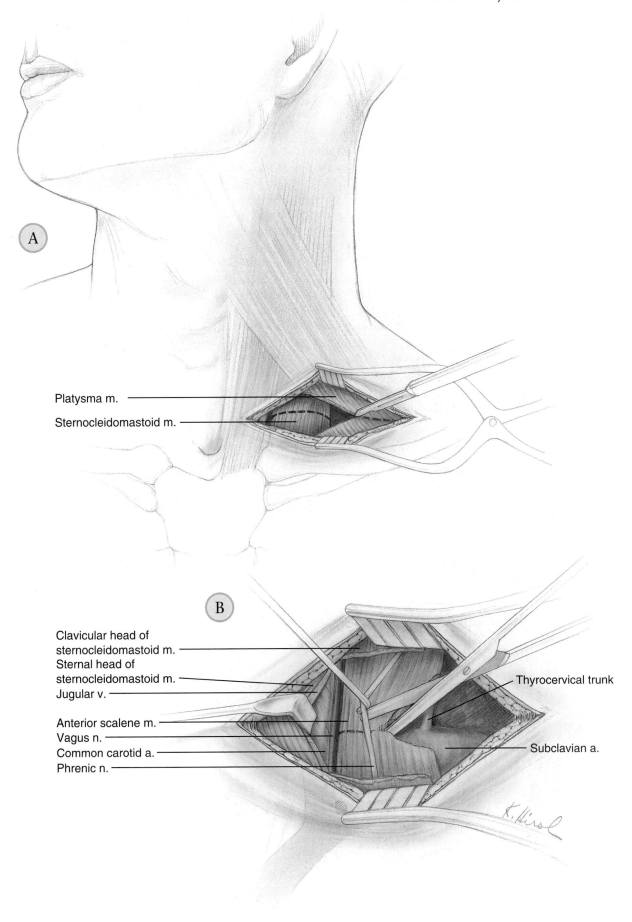

A

Platysma m.

Sternocleidomastoid m.

B

Clavicular head of
sternocleidomastoid m.
Sternal head of
sternocleidomastoid m.
Jugular v.

Anterior scalene m.
Vagus n.
Common carotid a.
Phrenic n.

Thyrocervical trunk

Subclavian a.

C

The subclavian artery is mobilized and the vertebral artery, internal mammary artery, and thyrocervical trunks are identified.

D

After systemic heparinization, the proximal subclavian artery is clamped, and the internal mammary artery is divided and ligated. Heifetz clips are placed on the vertebral artery and thyrocervical trunk, and the distal subclavian artery is clamped.

E

The proximal stump of the subclavian artery is oversewn with nonabsorbable monofilament vascular suture. The distal subclavian artery is mobilized to the common carotid artery, and a suitable place for anastomosis is selected. The common carotid artery is cross-clamped, and a longitudinal arteriotomy is made. An end-to-side anastomosis of the subclavian artery to the common carotid artery is then performed using continuous monofilament 5–0 or 6–0 suture. The anastomosis is begun in the center of the posterior wall, runs in both directions along the back wall from the inside, and is completed on the anterior wall. Before completion of the suture line, the carotid should be flushed in both directions to evacuate air and any debris. Flow should be established to the subclavian artery before establishing flow to the distal carotid artery to further guard against cerebral embolization.

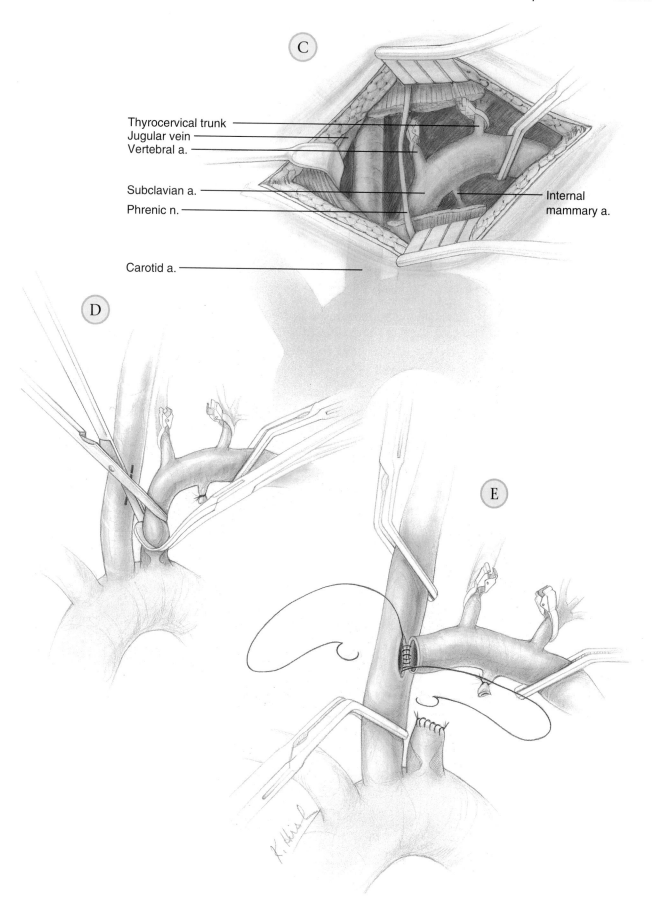

Thyrocervical trunk

Jugular vein

Vertebral a.

Subclavian a.

Phrenic n.

Internal mammary a.

Carotid a.

The subclavian artery is exposed through a supraclavicular incision in the neck as previously described. After division of the anterior scalene muscle, the common carotid artery is dissected slightly higher than for a direct carotid subclavian anastomosis in the neck. A suitable segment of subclavian artery distal to the thyrocervical trunk is selected for anastomosis. After application of the vascular clamps, a longitudinal arteriotomy is made in the subclavian artery and a vascular graft is sutured end-to-side using continuous 6–0 monofilament vascular suture. A variety of grafts may be selected including saphenous vein, polytetrafluoroethylene, or Dacron. It is our preference to use polytetrafluoroethylene for most cases because vein grafts may kink in this area.

After completion of the subclavian anastomosis, vascular clamps are removed from the subclavian artery, and the graft is allowed to fill with blood. The orientation and course of the graft at the base of the neck can then be visualized. Choosing an appropriate location for the carotid anastomosis and tailoring the proper length of graft are most important to avoid kinking of the graft when the neck is turned. Clamps are applied to the carotid artery and a longitudinal arteriotomy is made on the lateral aspect of the carotid artery. The bypass graft is anastomosed to the common carotid artery in an end-to-side fashion using continuous 5–0 or 6–0 monofilament suture. The anastomosis is begun in the center of the back wall, and the suture is run in both directions along the back wall from the inside.

Care must be taken to avoid too long an arteriotomy on either the carotid and subclavian anastomoses because this may result in kinking at the anastomosis. This problem is more likely when pliant saphenous veins are used.

Carotid subclavian bypasses that are too long can kink in the center when turning the neck. This results in poor flow and a tendency to thrombose.

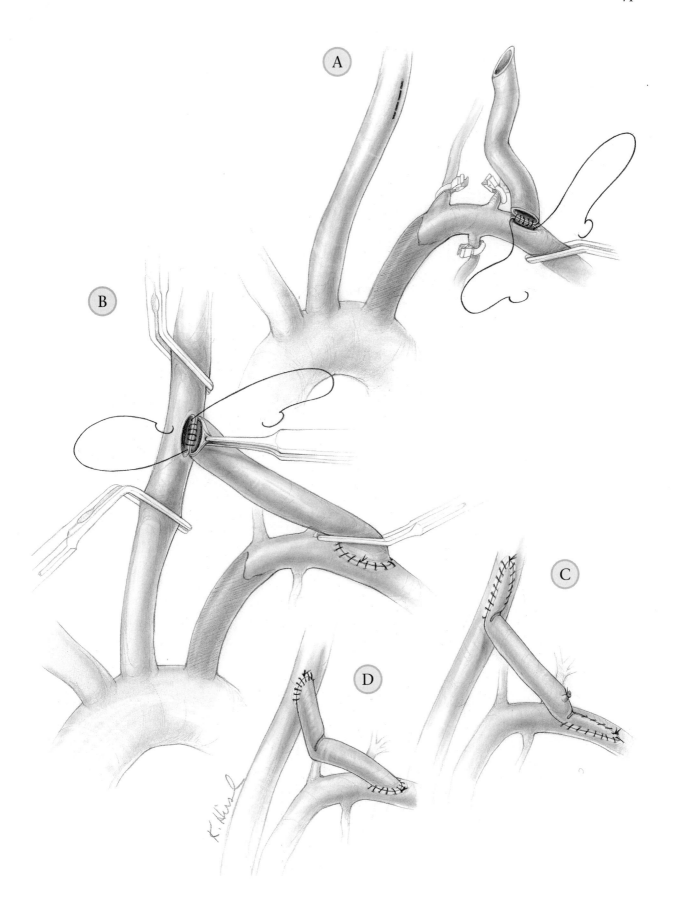

Patients with vertebral basilar ischemia caused by vertebral artery obstruction may benefit from vertebral artery revascularization. Such patients usually have occlusion or hypoplasia of one vertebral artery and severe stenosis in the contralateral vertebral artery. The vertebral artery can be revascularized by endarterectomy, interposition bypass, or reimplantation into the common carotid artery. Implantation of the vertebral artery into the common carotid artery is our procedure of choice.

(A) Patients must be evaluated with complete angiography including views of the aortic arch and intracranial circulation. Focal lesions of the orifice of the vertebral artery are most amenable to treatment. The proximal subclavian artery is exposed through a transverse supraclavicular incision with division of the anterior scalene muscle (see description on pages 41–43).

(B) Once the anterior scalene muscle is divided, the critical anatomy is evident. The phrenic nerve is protected from injury, and the thyrocervical trunk laterally and the origin of the vertebral artery are identified. The vertebral vein, which is immediately anterior to the artery, should be ligated and divided. Care should also be taken to avoid injury to the sympathetic ganglion lying slightly medial to the vertebral artery. SCM, Sternocleidomastoid.

(C) Endarterectomy of the orifice of the vertebral artery may be feasible for lesions limited to the vertebral origin. Vascular clamps are applied to the subclavian artery and its branches, and an arteriotomy is made in the subclavian artery opposite the orifice of the vertebral artery. An endarterectomy is performed with removal of the localized atheroma. This procedure is only rarely performed because most atherosclerotic plaques are extensive and involve long segments of the subclavian artery. If local endarterectomy is not followed by excellent back bleeding from a widely patent vertebral orifice, plans to endarterectomize should be abandoned. The subclavian artery should be closed primarily or with a patch graft, and alternate vertebral revascularization should be carried out.

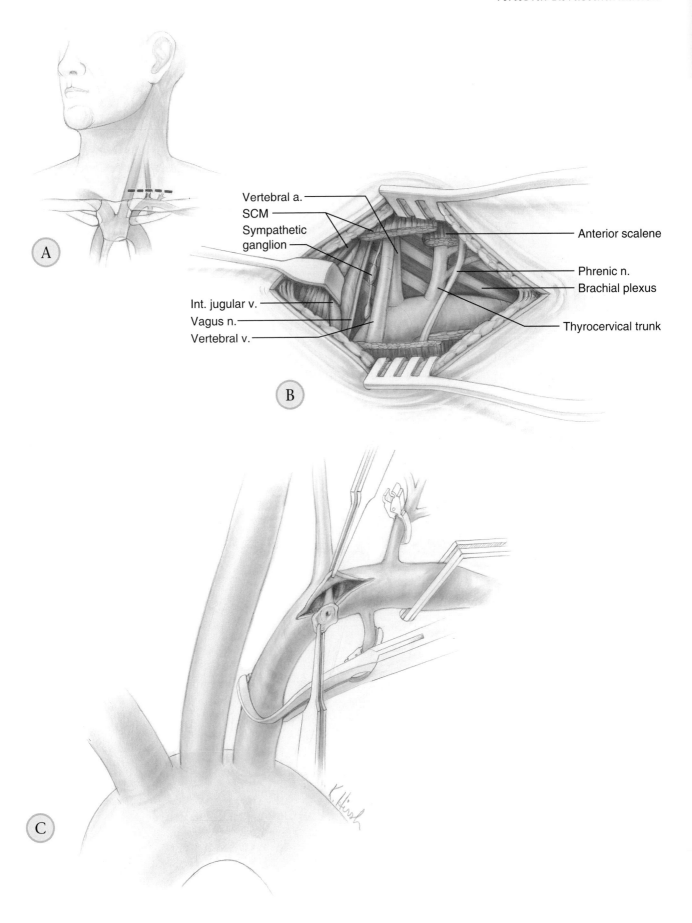

A

Vertebral a.
SCM
Sympathetic
ganglion

Anterior scalene

Phrenic n.
Brachial plexus

Int. jugular v.
Vagus n.
Vertebral v.

Thyrocervical trunk

B

C

(D) Implantation of the vertebral artery into the common carotid artery is the most widely used technique. Exposure of the subclavian, vertebral, and common carotid arteries is accomplished as described on pages 41–43. The vertebral artery is divided at its origin from the subclavian artery, and the proximal segment is oversewn. A suitable site for implantation into the carotid artery is selected. The carotid artery is clamped and a small 3-mm arteriotomy is made in the posterolateral aspect of the common carotid artery with an aortic punch.

(E) The vertebral artery is not widely spatulated, but anastomosed end-to-side into the common carotid artery with continuous 6–0 monofilament vascular suture. Medially rotating the carotid artery will assist in exposure.

(F) With a carotid anastomosis located on the lateral and posterior portion of the common carotid artery, the vertebral artery lies in a nonkinked position.

(G) If the common carotid artery is occluded or if one wishes to avoid even temporary cross-clamping of the carotid artery (i.e., contralateral carotid occlusion), reimplantation of the vertebral artery cannot be performed. Under these circumstances, the vertebral artery can be anastomosed to the distal subclavian artery using an interposition saphenous vein bypass. The vein is first anastomosed end-to-end to the vertebral artery and then implanted end-to-side to a suitable portion of the distal subclavian artery.

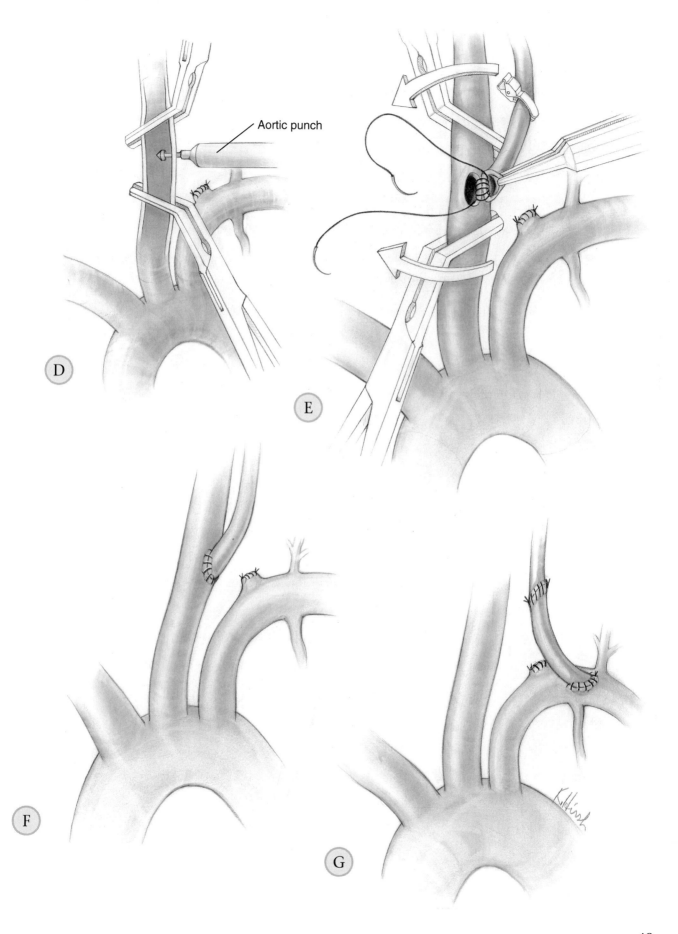

Aortic punch

D

E

F

G

Patients with innominate artery lesions may be treated with endarterectomy or arch bypass. Focal lesions of the origin of the innominate artery are best treated with endarterectomy, whereas extensive lesions are treated with bypasses from the ascending aorta to the carotid or subclavian artery or cross-neck bypasses such as carotid–subclavian or subclavian–subclavian bypasses.

For an innominate endarterectomy the patient is positioned and prepared for a median sternotomy. An incision is made from the suprasternal notch to the xiphoid process, and the sternum is divided in its midportion using a sternal saw.

The innominate vein is identified and mobilized. The anterior jugular vein is divided and ligated as it enters the innominate vein. The innominate vein is retracted inferiorly, and the underlying aortic arch is exposed. The innominate artery is identified and mobilized. Control is obtained of the distal innominate artery, and its junction to the aortic arch is dissected free. The origin of the left common carotid artery is identified.

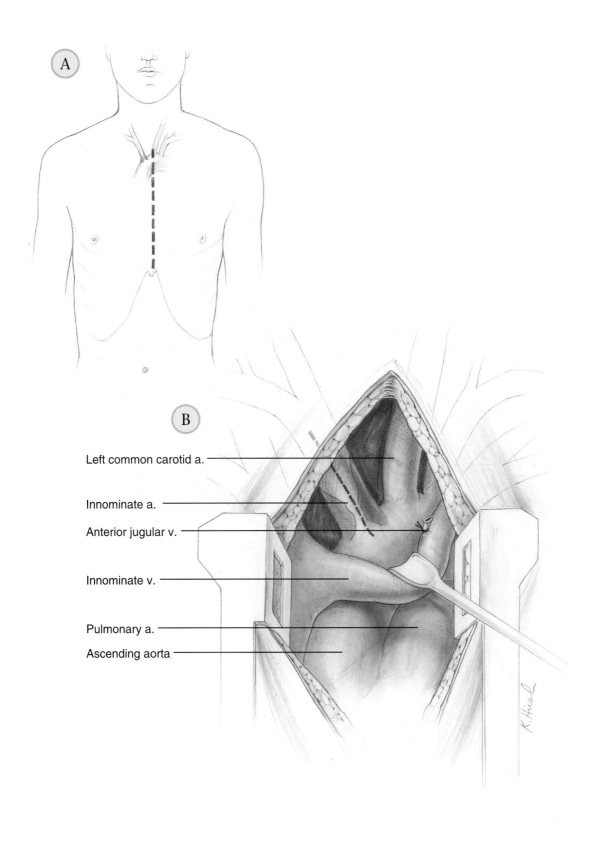

Left common carotid a.

Innominate a.

Anterior jugular v.

Innominate v.

Pulmonary a.

Ascending aorta

Separate control of the common carotid and subclavian artery can be obtained if necessary for distal control. Care should be exercised to avoid injury to the recurrent larnygeal nerve as it courses around the origin of the subclavian artery. After systemic heparinization the origin of the innominate artery is occluded with a narrow curved vascular clamp. This clamp should be carefully selected so that it extends onto the aortic arch for approximately one third of its circumference and yet does not occlude the orifice of the left common carotid artery. Clamps are applied to the distal innominate or the right carotid and subclavian arteries. A longitudinal arteriotomy is made in the innominate artery, and the atherosclerotic plaque is identified.

 Using an endarterectomy spatula, an endarterectomy is performed in the usual fashion, separating the intimal plaque from the underlying media and adventitia. The plaque is carefully dissected proximally and must be sharply divided within the aortic arch because innominate lesions are usually contiguous with aortic arch atheromas. The endarterectomized surface is carefully inspected to ensure that there is no loose debris.

 The arteriotomy is closed primarily with continuous 4–0 monofilament cardiovascular suture. On occasion, this arteriotomy may be closed with a patch, but this is usually not necessary.

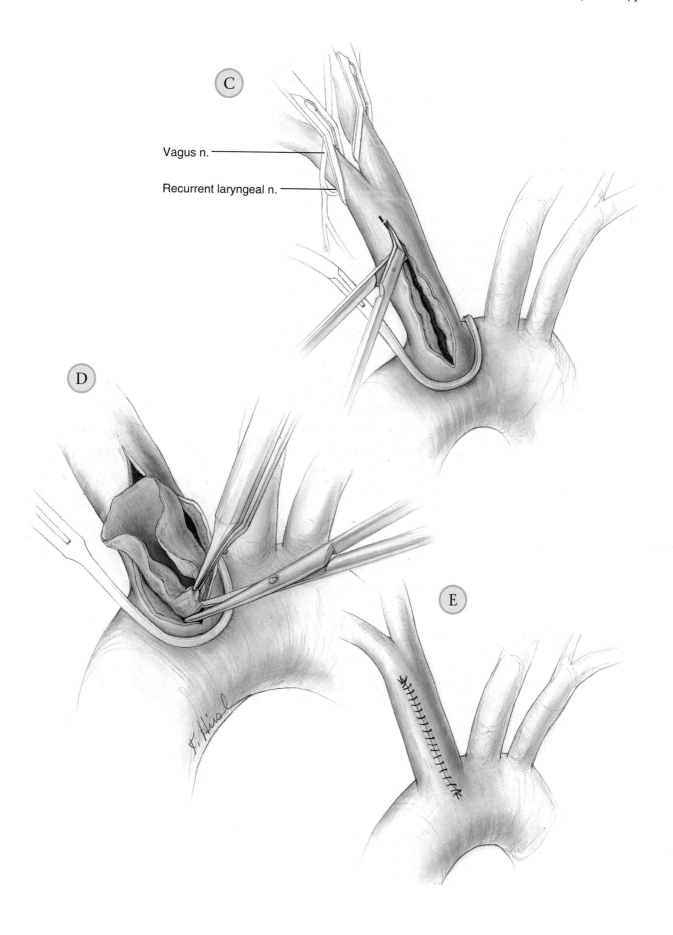

Vagus n.

Recurrent laryngeal n.

C

D

E

If the origin of the left carotid artery is quite close to the origin of the innominate artery, it may be impossible to place a clamp on the aortic arch without effectively occluding both carotid arteries. Endarterectomy may also be deemed unsuitable if the aortic arch is highly calcified such that safe clamping cannot be carried out. In these instances, bypass grafting allows the surgeon to choose the least diseased portion of the arch as the origination site. This usually is the more proximal portion of the arch inside the pericardium. As shown, a LeMole clamp is carefully placed on the arch. Close communication between the surgeon and anesthesiologist is required because systemic blood pressure should be decreased during clamping to provide secure clamp application and to avoid injury to the oft-diseased aorta. Satisfactory clamp occlusion is tested by first placing a small needle in the clamped portion of the aorta, and the arteriotomy is then carried out.

Depending on the size of the distal innominate artery, an 8- to 10-mm Dacron graft is selected and sewn in an end-to-side fashion to the aortic arch and in an end-to-end fashion to the transected distal innominate artery. Before completion of the closure, back flushing of any debris and air is accomplished and flow is restored first to the right subclavian and then to the right common carotid artery.

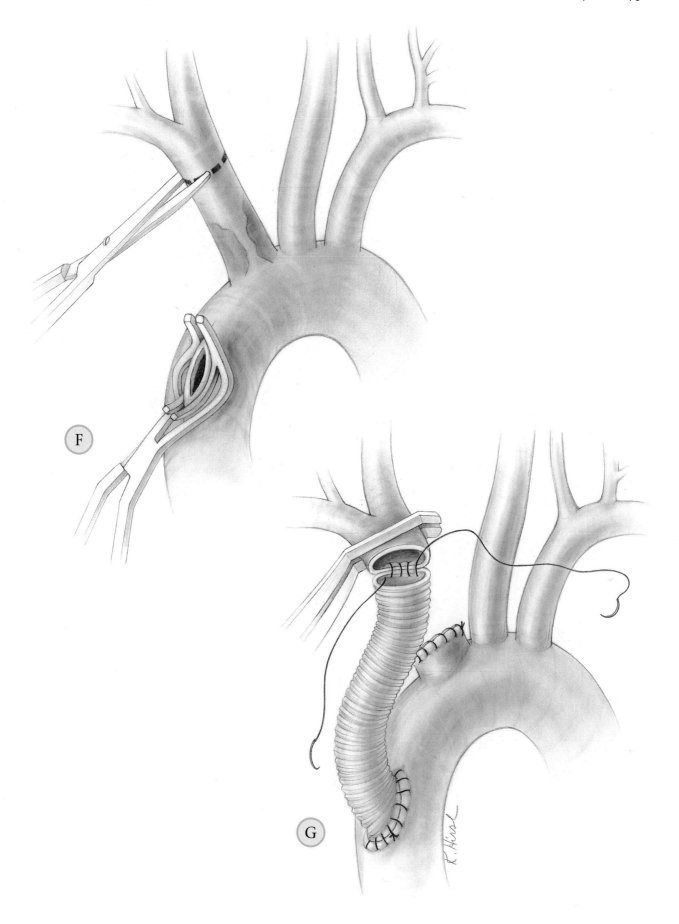

SECTION II

Treatment of Aneurysmal Disease

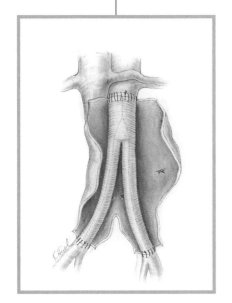

Aneurysms are the most dramatic manifestation of artery wall degeneration with arterial enlargement and possible sudden rupture, resulting in exsanguinating hemorrhage. Aneurysms may develop in any artery, but are most often found in the infrarenal abdominal aorta, which accounts for more than 80% of all aneurysms. Clinically significant aneurysms also occur in the thoracic and thoracoabdominal aorta, iliac arteries, femoral and popliteal arteries, carotid and visceral arteries. Although aneurysms have been noted since antiquity, effective treatment has been available for only the last 50 years. The first successful open aortic aneurysm repair was performed in 1951 by Norman Freeman using an autogenous iliac vein graft, followed shortly thereafter by Charles Dubost who used an aortic homograft to replace the aneurysm. The effectiveness of open surgical repair of aneurysms of all types stimulated the rapid growth and development of the field of vascular surgery. Durable synthetic fabric grafts were developed together with monofilament sutures, atraumatic vascular clamps, specialized instruments, lighting and magnification. Improvements in anesthesia, fluid management, and perioperative care progressively improved surgical results over the last three decades, establishing open surgical repair as the standard of care for patients with abdominal aortic aneurysms. About 10 years ago, a new concept in the treatment of aortic aneurysms was introduced: endovascular aortic aneurysm repair. This minimally invasive, endoluminal approach has reduced the magnitude of the operation with reduced patient morbidity and more rapid patient recovery. The techniques of endoluminal repair and perfection of endoluminal devices for the abdominal and thoracic aorta are still evolving, but the principles of endovascular repair (see later in this chapter) have become an essential part of vascular surgery.

Overview of Aneurysmal Disease

Aortic aneurysms are the thirteenth leading cause of death in the United States with 15,000 deaths from rupture per year. Over the last 30 years, the incidence of aortic aneurysms has increased fourfold, from 9 per 1,000 to 37 per 1,000 population, whereas deaths from heart attacks and strokes have decreased 30% to 40% over the same period. The prevalence of aneurysms increases with age, and an aneurysm is eight times more likely to develop in a man than a woman. Approximately 1 in 10 men 75 years or older will have an abdominal aortic aneurysm on ultrasound surveillance studies. Although aneurysms are more commonly found in men, the incidence of aneurysms in women older than 80 years approaches that in men. Women with aneurysms are more likely to sustain rupture and die of their aneurysm than men.

Most patients with aneurysms have risk factors for atherosclerosis and have evidence of atherosclerotic plaques in their coronary arteries, carotid or peripheral arteries. The relationship between aortic aneurysms and atherosclerosis has long been recognized, and abdominal aneurysms are usually referred to as "atherosclerotic aneurysms." However, a causal relation between atherosclerosis and aneurysm formation has not been proven. Multiple factors have been implicated in aneurysm pathogenesis including atherosclerosis, inflammation, and genetic predisposition, as well as localized activity of proteolytic enzymes and their inhibitors. The most prominent histologic finding in aneurysmal aortic walls is degeneration of the medial lamellar architecture with prominent loss of elastin. Adventitial inflammatory cells are often present, and increased proteolytic enzyme activity has been documented, stimulating research to develop inhibitors of proteolytic activity to prevent aneurysmal enlargement. Approximately 10% to 15% of patients with aneurysm have a family history of aneurysm, and aneurysms can be found in up to 30% of siblings of patients with aneurysm, suggesting genetic predisposition in many patients.

Aneurysms are usually asymptomatic and may be found as a pulsatile abdominal mass on physical examination. However, in patients with abdominal obesity, even large aneurysms may not be palpable. Abdominal ultrasound is the procedure of choice to image and diagnose aneurysms and to determine aneurysm size. Aneurysms may also be discovered as incidental findings on computed tomography (CT) or magnetic resonance (MR) imaging performed for other indications. Contrast CT scanning is the best imaging study to precisely define aneurysm size and shape and to plan appropriate treatment. CT scanning can determine if an aneurysm is leaking or ruptured and can define the characteristics of the nonaneurysmal aortic neck and iliac arteries to determine whether a patient is a candidate for endovascular aneurysm repair. Improvements in contrast CT and MR imaging with three-dimensional (3D) reconstruction have largely replaced angiography in the evaluation of aortic aneurysms. Angiography may not delineate aneurysm size accurately, due to the presence of mural thrombus in the aneurysm.

The natural history of aneurysms is to enlarge and rupture. Approximately 50% of patients with untreated aneurysms will die of rupture. The mortality of aortic aneurysm rupture is high, with more than half of patients dying suddenly before reaching medical help. Some patients develop severe pain and have contained ruptures providing the opportunity for emergent open surgical repair. The mortality rate for repair of ruptured aortic aneurysms is 50% to 90%. Therefore, every effort should be made to treat patients with aortic aneurysms on an elective basis to prevent rupture. Risk factors for rupture include aneurysm size, sex, hypertension, and chronic obstructive pulmonary disease (COPD), with the most dominant and important risk factor for rupture being aneurysm size. The annual risk for rupture of aneurysms less than 5 cm in diameter is 1% to 2%, while the risk for rupture of aneurysms 5 to 6 cm in diameter is approximately 10%, and the risk for rupture for aneurysms greater than 6 cm is 25% or more. Although large aneurysms are much more likely to rupture than small aneurysms, small aneurysms can and do rupture on occasion. The exact size at which an asymptomatic small abdominal aneurysm should be treated remains unsettled and has been the subject of two prospective randomized clinical trials of patients with aneurysms less than 5.5 cm. Patients who were randomized to ultrasound surveillance underwent open surgical repair if the aneurysm enlarged, became symptomatic, or ruptured. Patients under surveillance had a 1-year risk for rupture of 1%, but more than two thirds of the patients in the surveillance group required open surgical repair during the 5-year follow-up period. Thus, although early operation for patients with small aneurysms is not necessary, most will ultimately require surgical treatment.

Open surgical repair is effective in preventing aneurysm rupture and can be performed with a low mortality rate in properly selected patients. Improvements in surgical techniques and patient care have reduced the overall mortality rate for elective open surgical repair of aortic aneurysms to approximately 5%. Many patients with aneurysms, however, are elderly and have multiple comorbidities including coronary artery disease, congestive heart failure, COPD, and renal failure. These comorbidities may significantly increase the mortality of open surgery and may exclude patients as candidates for elective open surgical repair. In these patients, endovascular aneurysm repair is a good alternative, because this procedure may be performed through groin incisions and does not require abdominal aortic exposure and aortic cross-clamp. However, only 50% of patients with abdominal aortic aneurysm have suitable morphology for endovascular repair using currently available devices. Thus, careful patient evaluation is required with morphologic and risk/benefit analysis to select the most suitable treatment for each patient.

Open Repair of Abdominal Aortic Aneurysms

Open surgical repair is effective in preventing aneurysm rupture and is the standard of care in the treatment of patients with aortic aneurysms. The principle of open surgical repair is exclusion of the aneurysm from the circulation by replacing it with a prosthetic graft. Aortic blood flow is controlled with proximal and distal clamps, and the graft is anastomosed to nonaneurysmal aorta with permanent monofilament sutures. These sutures anchor the graft in place and provide permanent fixation of the fabric graft to the vessels. There is no substantial tissue healing of the fabric to the aorta, and long-term success of open surgical repair is dependent on continuing integrity of the anastomotic suture line.

Open repair may be performed through a transabdominal or retroperitoneal exposure of the aorta. Operative mortality rate ranges from 2% to 8% with mortality rates of approximately 5% in most current large multicenter experiences. Mortality rates of 1% to 2% can be achieved in young patients at low risk with minimal comorbidities, rapid postoperative recovery, and good long-term results. Older patients with cardiac, pulmonary, and renal disease may have operative mortality rates of 8% to 15% or greater. Major morbidity rates of 15% to 30% can be expected, and older patients may require postoperative rehabilitation and have prolonged recovery times.

Late complications of open aneurysm repair include anastomotic pseudoaneurysms, graft thrombosis, graft infection, aortoenteric fistulas, aneurysm rupture, colonic ischemia, and peripheral embolism. These complications may occur in 5% to 10% of patients. Reoperations for graft complications has a significantly greater mortality rate than primary elective aneurysm repair.

The 5-year survival rate of patients after successful elective aortic aneurysm repair is 60% to 70% with a 10-year survival rate of approximately 40%. Long-term survival of patients with aneurysm is less than age- and sex-matched patients without aneurysms. The increased mortality is mainly due to manifestations of atherosclerosis, particularly coronary artery disease. The causes of late death after aortic aneurysm reconstruction are cardiac disease (36–44%), cancer (15–25%), rupture of another aneurysm (8–11%), stroke (7–9%), and pulmonary disease (6–15%). Age, cardiac disease, carotid disease, renal disease, aneurysm extent, suprarenal extension, and external iliac involvement have been found to be independent risk factors predictive of late mortality after elective aortic aneurysm reconstruction.

Abdominal aortic aneurysms may be repaired through a transperitoneal or retroperitoneal approach. The retroperitoneal approach to the aorta (see page 79) is useful in patients with dense intraabdominal adhesions, colostomies, marked obesity, or other contraindications to a transperitoneal approach. Because control of the right common iliac artery may be more difficult with the retroperitoneal approach, we prefer transperitoneal exposure through a vertical midline or infraumbilical transverse incision in most patients.

The peritoneal bands binding the duodenum to the aneurysm are incised, and the parietal peritoneum is divided up to the ligament of Treitz. The duodenum is mobilized and retracted laterally. The retroperitoneum overlying the neck of the aneurysm is divided. The renal vein is identified and carefully dissected to expose the underlying neck of the aneurysm. When identified, prominent lymphatics are ligated. The retroperitoneal incision is carried down toward the aortic bifurcation slightly toward the vena caval side of the aneurysm. This avoids injury to the inferior mesenteric artery and its primary branches.

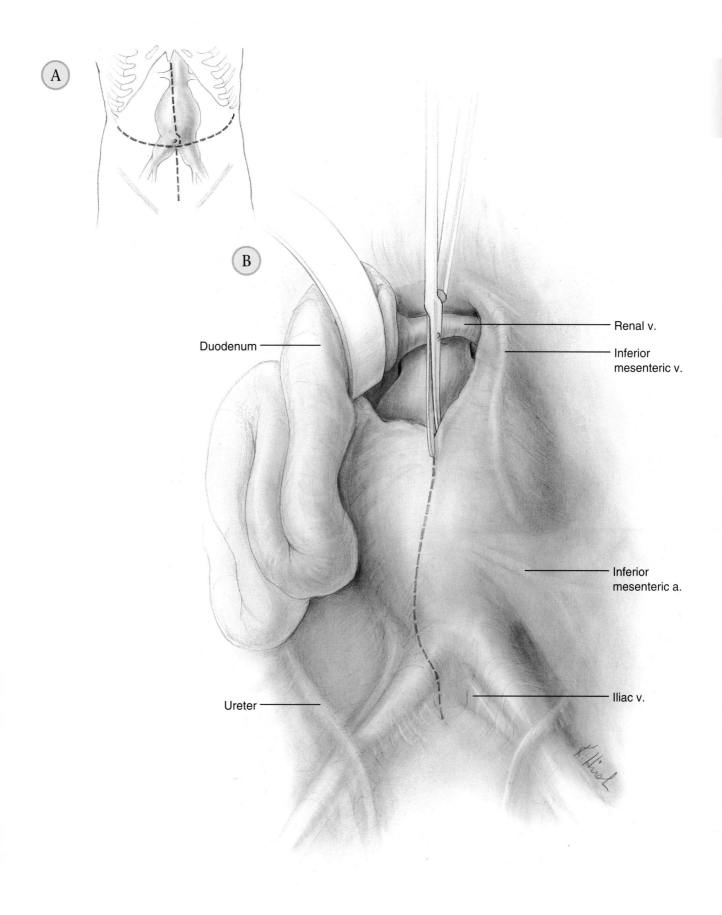

A

B

Duodenum

Renal v.

Inferior
mesenteric v.

Inferior
mesenteric a.

Ureter

Iliac v.

The left renal vein is mobilized and gently retracted superiorly. The renal arteries lie cephalad and posterior to the left renal vein. Mobilization of the vein protects the arteries from injury and greatly facilitates exposure of the rarely aneurysmal infrarenal segment of the aorta. When resecting a large aneurysm or one with a very short infrarenal neck, it may be necessary to divide and ligate the left renal vein to facilitate exposure of this infrarenal aortic segment. The vein should be divided in its midportion to preserve the gonadal and adrenal veins, which provide satisfactory venous outflow from the left kidney. A moistened umbilical tape or Penrose drain may be passed behind the aorta. Manipulation of the aneurysm itself should be assiduously avoided to minimize the risk for embolization of mural thrombus or atheromatous debris. Control of the iliac arteries is obtained distal to the aneurysm using minimal dissection to avoid injury to the iliac veins.

A Dacron graft equal in diameter to the infrarenal aorta is selected. If a knitted Dacron graft is used, blood is withdrawn from the vena cava to preclot the graft. Heparin (100 U/k) is administered intravenously, and the infrarenal aorta is cross-clamped. In this example of an infrarenal aneurysm limited to the aorta itself, minimal dissection of the common iliac arteries is required. Angled vascular clamps can be applied to these vessels without the necessity for circumferential control. Clamps must avoid injury to the ureters and underlying iliac veins and should be placed so as to avoid fracturing atherosclerotic plaques. To decrease blood loss, a small vascular clamp can be placed on the proximal inferior mesenteric artery. The aortic aneurysm is incised with heavy scissors.

Intraluminal mural thrombus is often extensive and should be removed.

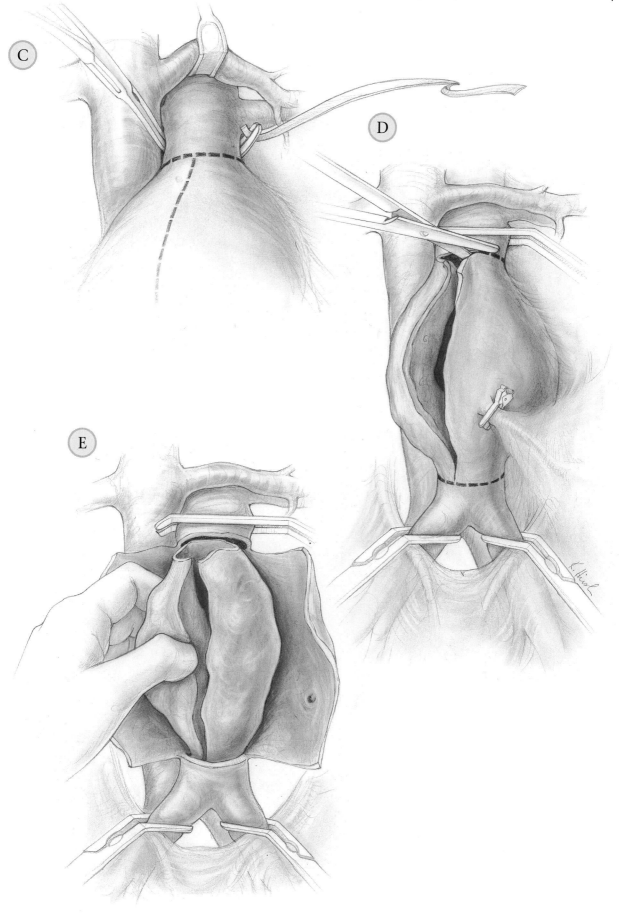

Back bleeding from lumbar arteries is controlled with deep "figure of eight" ligatures of stout, nonabsorbable suture. If the inferior mesenteric artery is occluded, it can be ignored. If pulsatile back bleeding is encountered, the vessel can be suture ligated from within the aneurysm with a figure of eight suture or ligated flush with its origin on the outside of the aneurysm. Atherosclerotic debris and any residual thrombus is carefully removed from the proximal and distal aorta at the site of anastomosis.

The Dacron graft is anastomosed to the infrarenal aorta using the endoaneurysmorrhaphy technique. A 3–0 nonabsorbable monofilament suture is passed through the graft and the posterior wall of the aorta. A wide and deep "bite" through the full thickness of the aortic wall including the intima, media, and adventitia is essential. The suture is tied and gentle traction is applied defining a "rim" of aorta at the suture line. This facilitates placement of the remaining back wall sutures from the inside of the aorta.

The anastomosis is continued along the posterior wall in both directions, placing large and deep sutures into the aorta. Uniform tension is maintained on the suture line by the assistant so that the graft remains firmly opposed to the aorta.

The continuous suture line is completed anteriorly and tied.

The integrity of the proximal suture line is checked by occluding the distal graft with the fingers and slowly releasing the proximal clamp. The posterior and anterior aspect of the suture line is carefully inspected. Leaks may be repaired with 4–0 or 5–0 suture, using pledgets if necessary. Preclotting of the graft is checked at this point. If the interstices of the Dacron graft are not fully sealed, intermittent release of the proximal clamp will complete the preclotting process in several minutes even with full heparinization. The distal anastomosis should not be performed until integrity of the proximal suture line and graft are ensured.

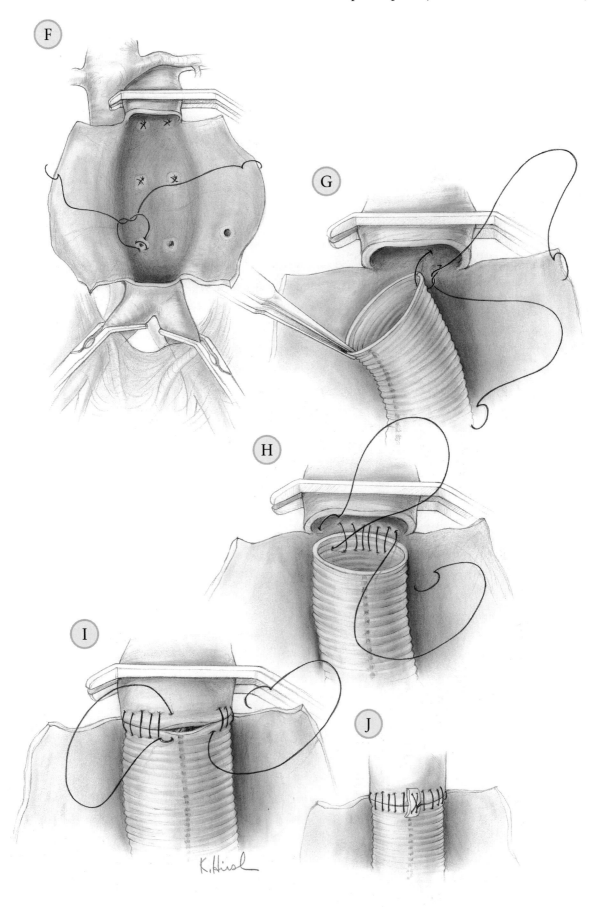

The Dacron "tube" graft is cut to appropriate length, and the distal anastomosis is performed. The suture line is begun in the center of the back wall through the inside of the aorta and run in both directions using 3–0 nonabsorbable monofilament suture. Before placement of the final sutures in the anterior wall, the aortic clamp and then the iliac artery clamps are opened to flush out any air, thrombus, or debris. After the distal suture has been tied, the iliac clamps are removed and the integrity of the distal suture line is checked. The proximal aortic clamp is then slowly released. During the first few pulses the assistant can compress the common femoral arteries in the groin to divert blood into the internal iliac arteries and prevent embolization to the lower extremities. If declamping hypotension is noted, the surgeon pinches the midportion of the graft, allowing every third or fourth pulse through until blood pressure greater than 100 mm Hg is maintained.

Systemic heparinization may be reversed at this time with 50 to 100 mg protamine. The aneurysm wall is closed over the Dacron graft using a continuous suture. The retroperitoneum is then reapproximated to provide a second layer of viable tissue between the duodenum and prosthetic graft. This greatly decreases the likelihood of an aortoduodenal fistula. In closing the pelvic retroperitoneum, care should be taken to avoid injury to the ureters.

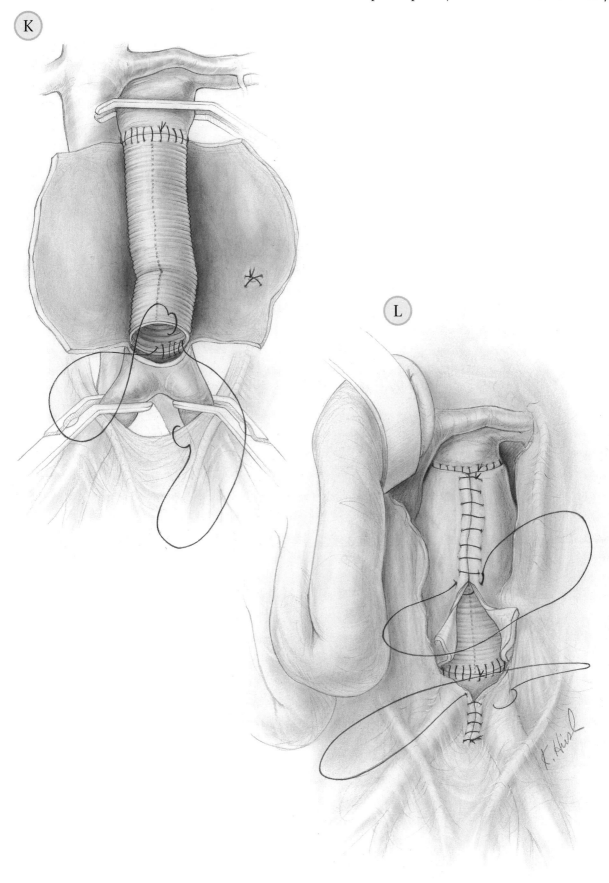

If aneurysmal disease extends to the common iliac arteries, a bifurcated graft is necessary (aortoiliac bypass). The iliac arteries are clamped distal to the aneurysm; this may require individual clamping of the internal and external iliac arteries. When dissecting at this level, the ureter should be identified and protected together with the pelvic autonomic nerves that pass lateral to medial at the junction of the left internal and external iliac arteries. To avoid injury to the nerves and postoperative impotence, it may be advisable not to incise along the left common iliac artery as shown but rather transect the distal common iliac artery at the *dotted line*.

The proximal aortic anastomosis is performed as previously described, except a bifurcated Dacron graft is selected. One limb of graft is then anastomosed to the nonaneurysmal common iliac artery in an end-to-end fashion using 4–0 nonabsorbable monofilament suture. This anastomosis may be performed using the endoaneurysmorrhaphy technique as shown, or the iliac artery may be completely divided and a standard end-to-end anastomosis performed. After completion of one iliac anastomosis, the distal iliac clamp is removed to retrograde fill the graft, flush out air and debris, and assess the integrity of the suture line. The iliac limb is then pinched and the proximal aortic clamp is released to flush out the aorta through the yet unattached graft limb. This limb is then clamped and flow is established to one leg. Heparinized saline is used to rinse the blood out of the unanastomosed limb to prevent thrombus formation. The second iliac anastomosis is then performed. Before completion of the anterior wall, the proximal and distal clamps are sequentially removed to flush the graft and clear it of air and debris. Systemic heparinization may be reversed with protamine, and the aneurysm wall is closed over the graft. The retroperitoneum is closed as described above.

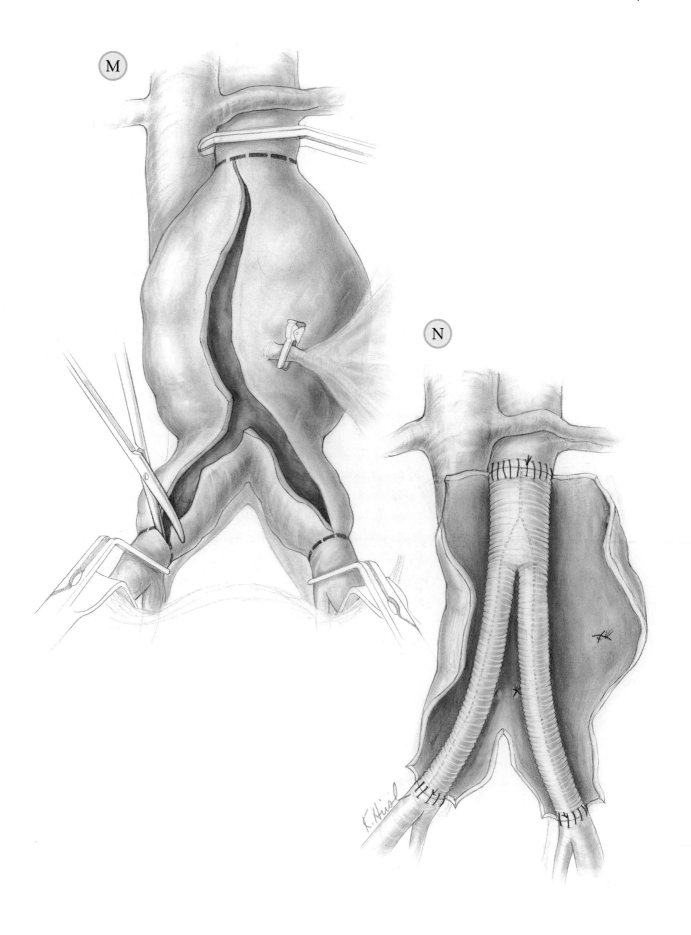

If an internal iliac aneurysm is present, it must be ligated to prevent rupture. This can be accomplished from within the aneurysm by extending the incision in the aneurysm and exposing the distal neck of the internal iliac artery aneurysm.

 The orifice of the distal internal iliac artery is oversewn from within the aneurysm, and the graft limb is anastomosed end-to-end to the external iliac artery. Spatulation of the external iliac artery by extending the arteriotomy on the anterior wall facilitates size matching and avoids atherosclerotic plaques that are frequently present at the iliac bifurcation.

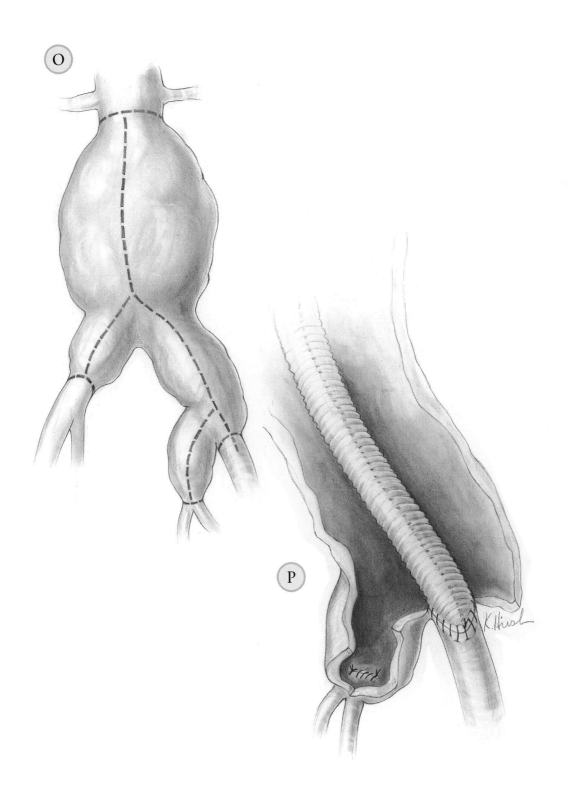

Revascularization of Inferior Mesenteric Artery

The inferior mesenteric artery provides blood flow to the sigmoid colon with added collateral supply from the superior mesenteric artery through branches of the middle colic artery and from the internal iliac artery through the superior hemorrhoidal arteries. The inferior mesenteric artery arises from the anterior wall of abdominal aortic aneurysms and is often occluded by mural thrombus within the aneurysm. In patients who have a patent inferior mesenteric artery and who have a normal superior mesenteric artery and patent internal iliac arteries, the inferior mesenteric artery can usually be safely ligated during aneurysm repair. However, in patients with superior mesenteric artery stenosis, internal iliac aneurysms or obstruction, or with compromised mesenteric collateral blood, such as may occur with prior intestinal surgery, revascularization of the inferior mesenteric artery should be considered. This is particularly true in patients who have a large and prominent inferior mesenteric artery demonstrated on preoperative imaging studies or found at the time of operation. Although colon infarction is uncommon after elective aortic aneurysm repair, it is a devastating postoperative complication that can be avoided by inferior mesenteric artery revascularization during aneurysm repair.

Strong consideration should be given to revascularization of the IMA at the time of aneurysm repair if (1) the superior mesenteric artery is obstructed; (2) previous intraabdominal operations have disturbed mesenteric collateral blood flow; or (3) the internal iliac arteries are obstructed or require ligation because of aneurysmal disease. Preoperative angiography with visualization of all three main visceral vessels (celiac, SMA, IMA) is most useful in making this decision. If a patent IMA is ligated during aneurysm repair, the sigmoid colon should be carefully inspected before abdominal closure to be certain that colon ischemia is not present. This is especially true after repair of a ruptured aneurysm.

(Q) Pulsatile back bleeding from the inferior mesenteric artery (IMA) orifice usually signifies adequate collateral blood flow. The IMA may be suture ligated from within the aneurysmal sac.

(R) If reimplantation of the inferior mesenteric artery (IMA) is indicated on the basis of preoperative angiography or intraoperative signs of inadequate colonic blood flow, the vessel can be reimplanted into the side of the aortic graft. Excision of a patch of aortic wall, surrounding the orifice of the IMA, and careful eversion endarterectomy of the vessel may be helpful. A button of the graft should be excised to match the size of the aortic patch.

(S) If the proximal inferior mesenteric artery (IMA) is extensively diseased or cannot readily be reimplanted into the Dacron graft, an interpositioned graft should be used to revascularize the IMA. A prosthetic graft or saphenous vein can be used.

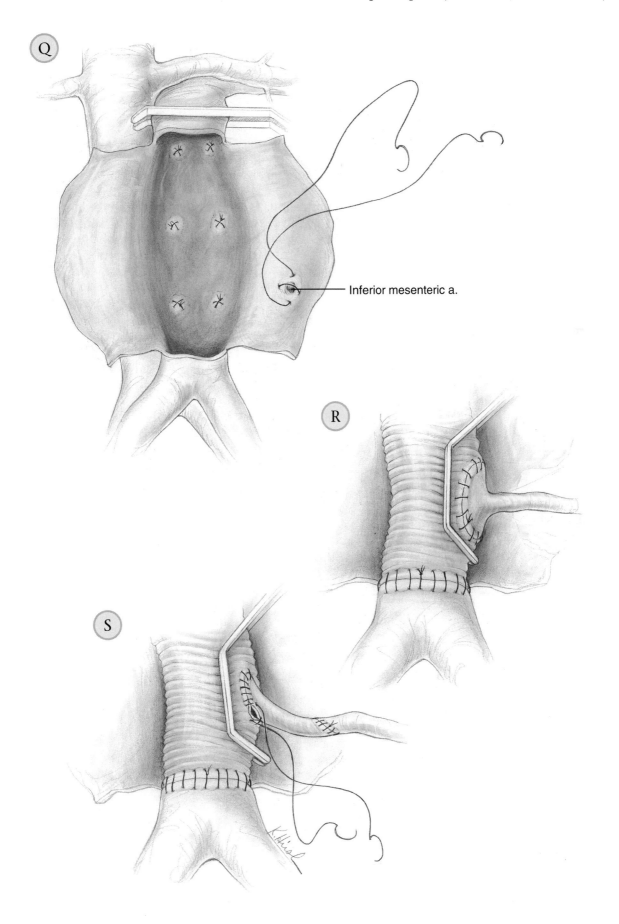

Inferior mesenteric a.

Horseshoe Kidney (Transperitoneal and Retroperitoneal Approaches)

Horseshoe kidney is a developmental anomaly in which the lower poles of the two kidneys are fused and lie on the anterior surface of the aorta. The prevalence rate of horseshoe kidney in the general population is 0.1% to 0.25%. Horseshoe kidneys commonly have multiple renal arteries with three or more renal arteries present in 80% of cases. In patients with aortic aneurysms, these multiple accessory renal arteries commonly arise from the aortic aneurysm and must be considered in undertaking aneurysm repair. Preoperative contrast CT scanning can confirm the presence of a horseshoe kidney and define the renal arteries with 3D reconstruction. Preoperative planning may be supplemented with angiography. Endovascular repair may be considered in patients with horseshoe kidney, but the presence of multiple accessory renal arteries often precludes this approach.

Horseshoe kidney is usually accompanied by downward displacement of the kidneys and anterior displacement of the ureters. Occasionally, a single ureter may drain the entire collecting system. The isthmus joining the lower poles of the kidneys may contain calyceal elements. Hence, division of the isthmus should be avoided to prevent the possibility of urinary leakage and subsequent graft infection. Usually, the isthmus can be mobilized and separated from the aneurysm, allowing the surgeon to work above and below the renal mass to gain proximal and distal control. If the isthmus is clearly a fibrous band, it can be divided.

Exposure may be obtained either transperitoneally through a vertical midline or transverse incision (see pages 60–61) or retroperitoneally (see page 79). The transperitoneal approach permits individual control of multiple renal arteries and better exposure of the right iliac artery. The retroperitoneal approach, posterior to the left kidney, avoids problems with the isthmus and collecting system but may make revascularization of accessory renal arteries and the right iliac artery more difficult. Reimplantation of accessory renal arteries can be performed from within the aneurysm using the technique used with thoracoabdominal aneurysm repair (see page 129). If necessary, the right iliac artery can be readily exposed using a right lower quadrant retroperitoneal incision.

In this case, the aorta is approached transperitoneally. Control of the neck of the aneurysm is achieved at the level of the left renal vein, and the iliac arteries are controlled distal to the aneurysm. The isthmus of the horseshoe kidney is separated from the aneurysm, and the two accessory renal arteries, exiting from the anterior wall of the aneurysm, are dissected. After systemic heparinization, the infrarenal aorta, iliac arteries, and accessory renal arteries are clamped. The aneurysm is opened leaving a button of aorta around the accessory renal arteries.

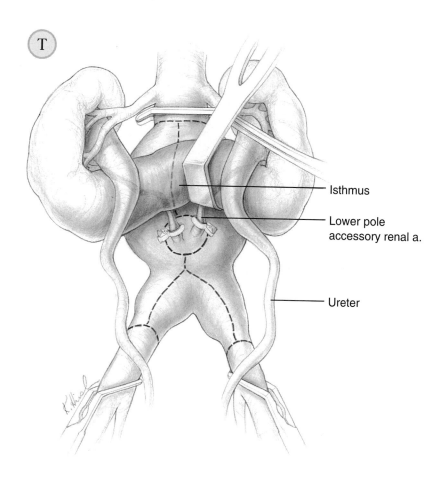

Isthmus

Lower pole
accessory renal a.

Ureter

The mural thrombus is removed from the aneurysm. Lumbar arteries and the orifice of the inferior mesenteric artery are oversewn from within the aneurysm. The proximal aorta anastomosis is performed using running 3–0 nonabsorbable monofilament suture. Gentle retraction of the isthmus inferiorly facilitates exposure for the proximal anastomosis. The Dacron graft is passed under the isthmus of the kidney within the aneurysmal sac to the iliac arteries.

 The isthmus of the kidney is retracted superiorly to facilitate the iliac anastomoses (see pages 69–71). After flushing the graft, unclamping the aorta, and revascularizing the lower extremities, a vascular clamp is placed on the side of the Dacron graft. An opening is made in the anterior wall of the graft at a suitable location, and the button of aorta containing the accessory renal arteries is anastomosed using 4–0 or 5–0 monofilament nonabsorbable suture. If it appears that the iliac anastomoses will be time consuming or it is necessary to carry the bifurcation graft to the femoral arteries, it is advisable to implant the renal arteries first to minimize renal ischemia time.

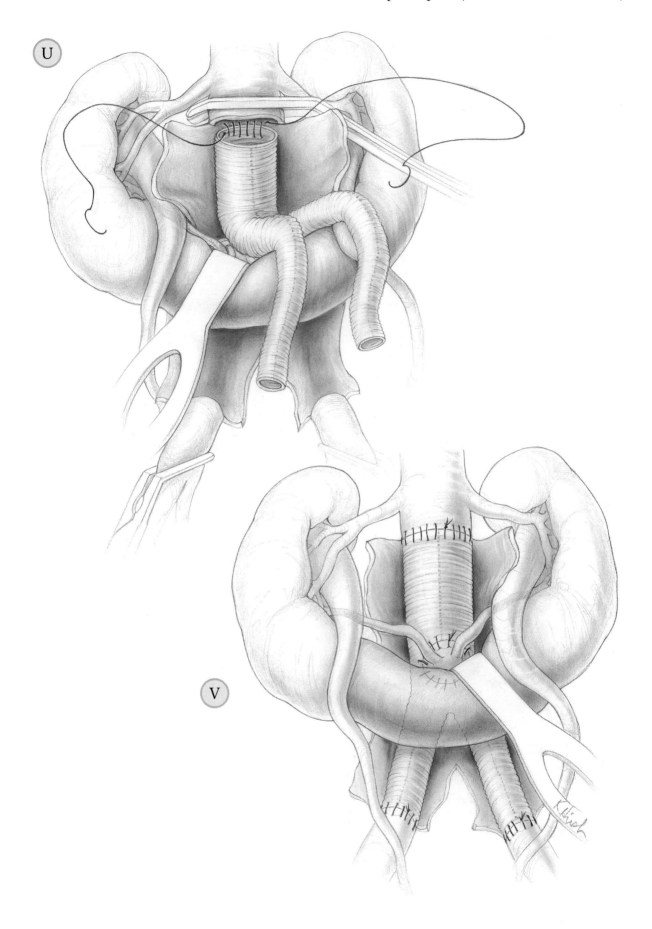

For retroperitoneal exposure, the patient is positioned on a bean bag, with the left shoulder elevated 45° and the left arm in a sling anteriorly. The hips are rotated approximately 20° to 30° and are as flat as possible to allow access to the right groin, if needed. A transverse incision is made from the tip of the twelfth rib to the midline 2 cm above or below the umbilicus. The external oblique, internal oblique, and transverse abdominus muscles are divided laterally. The anterior rectus sheath, left rectus abdominal muscle, and posterior rectus sheath are divided, leaving the peritoneum intact. The peritoneum is mobilized to the right with visualization of the iliopsoas muscle and ureter.

Retroperitoneal exposure of the aorta can be obtained in the plane anterior or posterior to the kidney. For procedures involving primarily the infrarenal aorta and iliac anteriors, we prefer the approach anterior to the kidney. For procedures involving the upper abdominal aorta, visceral arteries, and renal arteries, we prefer the retrorenal plane with mobilization of the left kidney anteriorly.

Retroperitoneal exposure of aortic aneurysm with horseshoe kidney in plane anterior to the kidney. The isthmus of the horseshoe kidney is anterior to the aneurysm and two accessory renal arteries arise from the anterior wall of the aneurysm. The urinary collecting system often crosses the isthmus of the horseshoe kidney, and division of the isthmus may result in urinary leak. Issues related to the horseshoe kidney may be avoided by mobilizing the kidney anteriorly and utilizing the retrorenal plane, as shown in Figure Z, page 81.

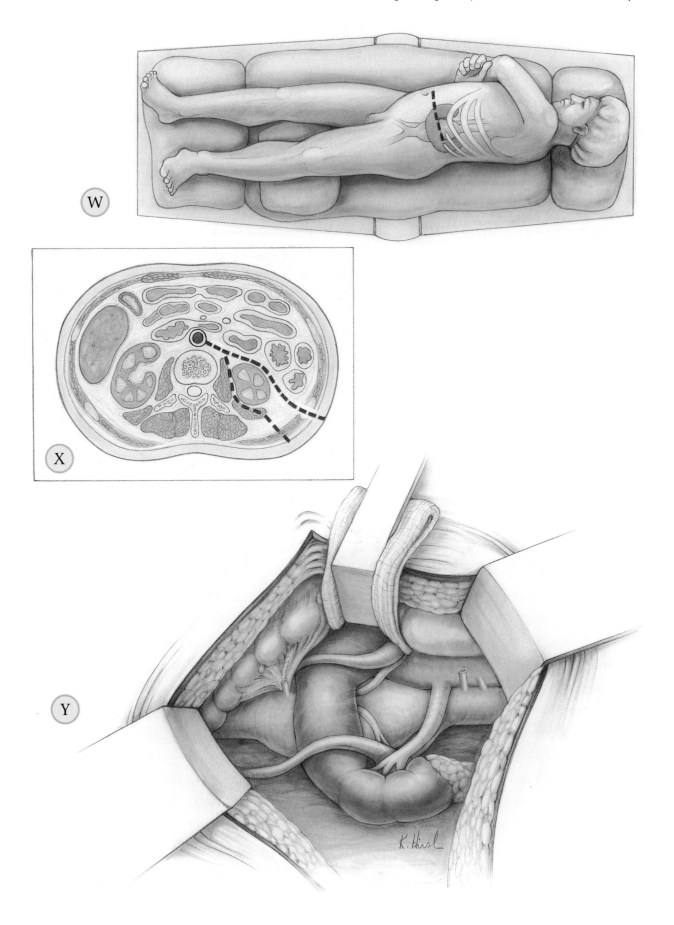

The horseshoe kidney is mobilized anteriorly, exposing the main left renal artery, which arises in the normal location above the aneurysm and the accessory renal arteries that arise from the anterior wall of the aneurysm. Control is obtained of the aortic neck below the main renal arteries as well as the distal aorta and iliac arteries. Following heparinization, the infrarenal aorta and distal aorta are clamped and the aneurysm is opened posterolaterally. Mural thrombosis is removed and lumbar arteries are oversewn.

A knitted polyester graft is anastomosed to the proximal and distal aorta using 3–0 or 4–0 polypropylene suture. An opening is made in the anterior wall of the prosthetic graft, and the accessory renal arteries are sutured to the graft from within the aneurysm using large through and through bites through the aneurysm wall. The inferior mesenteric artery may be anastomosed to the prosthetic graft in a similar fashion if it is of large caliber or has poor backbleeding. In this case, the inferior mesenteric artery was occluded and was suture ligated. The aneurysm wall is then closed over the prosthetic graft using 3–0 polypropylene suture.

Artist's rendition of completed repair after kidney is returned to its normal retroperitoneal location. For retrorenal approach and repair, surgical exposure as shown in this drawing is not needed.

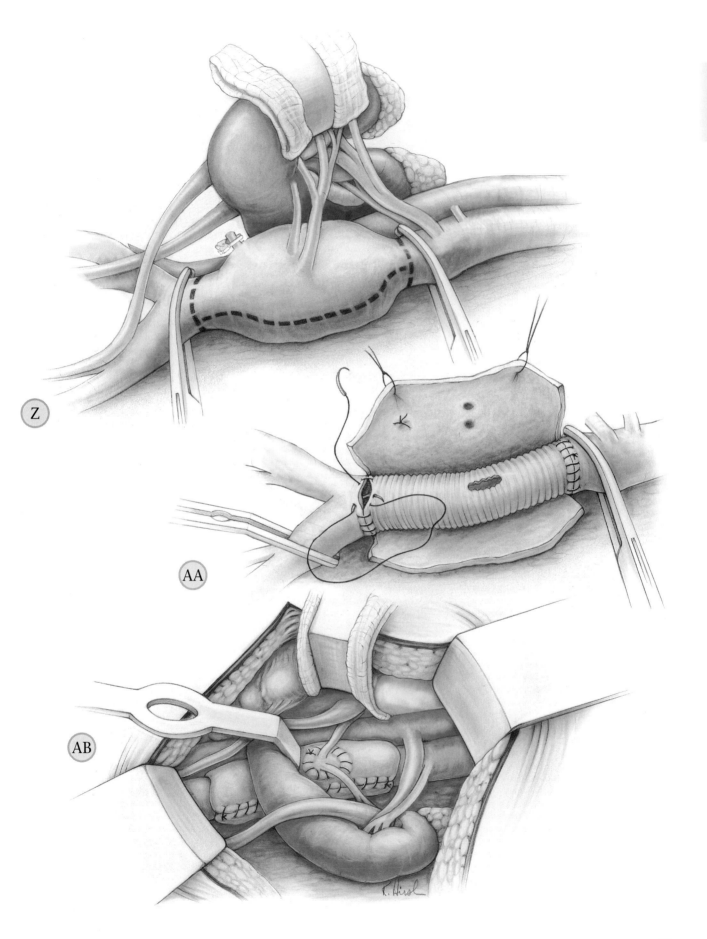

Open Repair of Juxtarenal Aortic Aneurysms

 Juxtarenal aortic aneurysm extending to the level of the renal arteries. There is no suitable infrarenal neck for clamping and anastomosis.

 The left renal vein is mobilized and retracted superiorly. Circumferential control of the suprarenal aorta and iliac arteries is obtained. Following systemic heparinization, the suprarenal aorta and the iliac arteries are clamped. The aneurysm is opened, mural thrombus is removed, and the lumbar arteries are oversewn. The posterior wall of the proximal aneurysm may be left intact, but we usually prefer to divide it for better visualization of the orifices of the renal arteries.

 A knitted polyester graft is saturated end-to-end to the juxtarenal aorta using running 3–0 or 4–0 polypropylene suture.

 The lower portion of the renal artery ostia may be included in the suture line for extra support.

The distal anastomosis is completed to the aortic bifurcation (as shown here) or to the iliac arteries in the case of an aortoiliac aneurysm. The inferior mesenteric artery is revascularized by anastomosing it to the anterior wall of the polyester graft using 6–0 polypropylene suture.

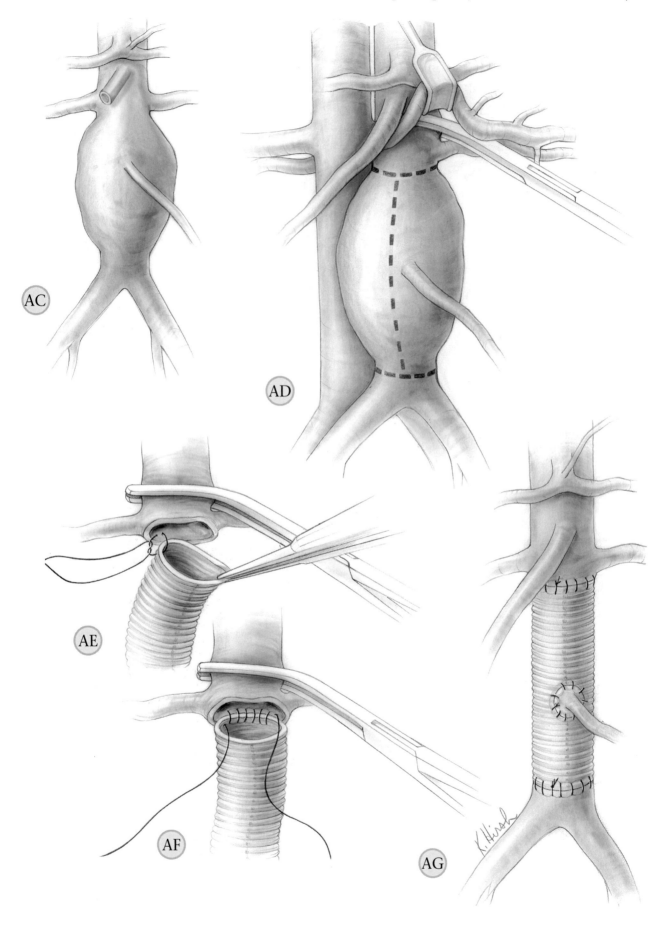

AC

AD

AE

AF

AG

K. Hirsh

Open Repair of Suprarenal Aortic Aneurysms

(AH) Aneurysm extending above the level of the renal arteries.

(AI) The supraceliac aorta is exposed through a transperitoneal approach for cross-clamp at this level.

(AJ) The aneurysm is opened, mural thrombus is removed, and lumbar arteries are over-sewn from within the aneurysm. Depending on the extent of the aneurysm, the proximal aorta may be divided to include or exclude the renal arteries in the primary aortic anastomosis. In this case, the right renal artery is divided, leaving a small cuff of aneurysm wall to facilitate anastomosis. The left renal artery and superior mesenteric artery remain attached to the proximal aorta.

(AK) A knitted polyester graft is sutured first to the proximal aorta and then to the distal aorta using 3–0 or 4–0 polypropylene suture. After restoring flow to the visceral branches and distal aorta, a partial occlusion clamp is applied to the prosthetic graft for right renal anastomosis. A small oval is removed from the polyester graft and the right renal artery is sutured to the graft using 5–0 polypropylene suture.

(AL) If both renal arteries arise from the suprarenal aneurysm, the proximal aortic anastomosis is to the nonaneurysmal aorta at the level of the superior mesenteric artery. After completion of the proximal and distal aortic anastomoses, each renal artery is separately reimplanted into the prosthetic aortic graft.

(AM) If the proximal renal artery is obstructed and cannot be readily opened with orifice endarterectomy, or if excess tension does not allow easy primary anastomosis to the aortic graft, we prefer 6-mm PTFE or Dacron polyester grafts.

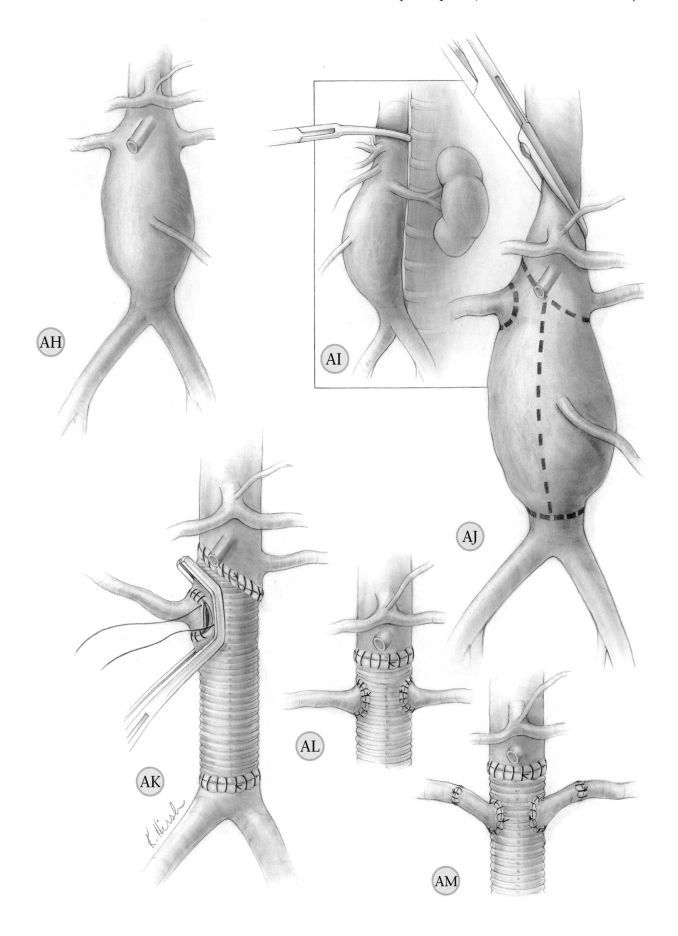

AH

AI

AJ

AK

K. Hirsch

AL

AM

Abdominal Aortic Aneurysm with Aortocaval Fistula

Occasionally, an abdominal aortic aneurysm may rupture or erode into the inferior vena cava or iliac veins resulting in an aortocaval fistula. Among patients with atherosclerotic abdominal aortic aneurysms, the incidence rate of aortocaval fistula is 0.2% to 1.3%. It has been suggested that adventitial inflammatory reaction around large aneurysms may encompass the vena cava and iliac veins, thus preventing free rupture in the event of aortic wall necrosis and rupture in the direction of the vein. This leaves no surgical plane between the aneurysm and vena cava. Approximately 5% to 10% of aortocaval fistulas occur in patients with mycotic aneurysms, Marfan's syndrome, or Ehlers-Danlos syndrome.

Patients with aortocaval fistula may present with acute right heart failure and venous engorgement. The symptoms may include hypotension, abdominal or low back pain, dyspnea, tachycardia, cardiomegaly, increased central venous pressure, pulmonary edema, and lower limb edema. Most patients have a palpable abdominal mass and an abdominal thrill with a loud machinery murmur. Preoperative clinical diagnosis of an aortocaval fistula may be confirmed with contrast CT scan, MR imaging, or ultrasound or aortography. The natural history of aortocaval fistula is cardiac decompensation and death, thus emergency repair is the only treatment option. The operative strategy is closure of the aortocaval fistula from within the aneurysm sac and repair of the aneurysm with a prosthetic graft. The operative mortality rate of emergent repair is high, approximately 30% to 40%, because of blood loss, cardiac decompensation, and pulmonary embolism. New endovascular strategies using transvenous occlusion balloons to obstruct the aortocaval fistula will facilitate open surgical control and repair. Endovascular repair using stent grafts may be used in suitable patients with favorable morphology demonstrated on preoperative imaging studies.

If the diagnosis of aortocaval fistula is known before surgery, particular care should be taken to obtain proximal and distal control of the aneurysm with the minimal amount of retroperitoneal dissection, mainly because lumbar and retroperitoneal veins are distended and can bleed copiously. The vena cava should not be dissected; in particular, no attempt should be made to separate the aneurysm from the vena cava because the two structures are densely adherent and dissection can result in extensive hemorrhage.

The aortocaval fistula is best controlled from within the aneurysm. After clamping the aorta and iliac arteries, the aneurysm is opened, mural thrombus is removed, and the fistula is controlled by compressing the vena cava with the fingers or sponge sticks as shown. The fistula can then be oversewn using large deep sutures through the wall of the aneurysm (see Fig. I).

Alternatively, a urinary catheter with a 30-ml balloon can be inserted into the fistula. Gentle traction allows hemostasis without continued obstruction of vena cava blood flow. This technique is usually satisfactory only for small fistulae.

Closure of the aortocaval fistula is from within the aneurysm using a continuous lateral suture. Hemostasis is obtained by proximal and distal compression using sponge sticks. After closure of the aortocaval fistula, replacement of the aneurysmal aorta with a Dacron graft is carried out as described in Section 1.

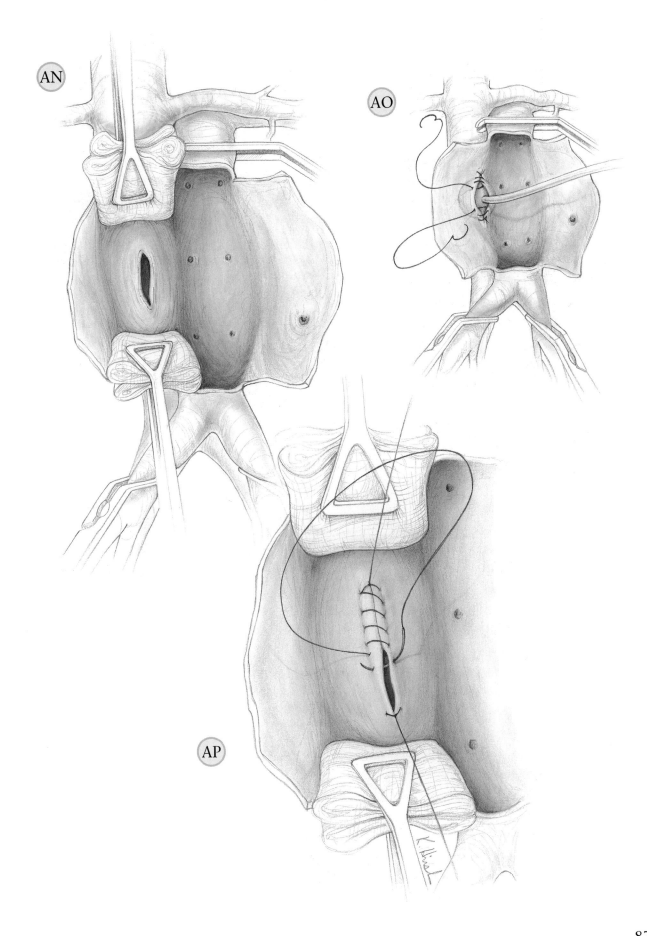

Overview of Endovascular Procedures

Transfemoral endoluminal abdominal aortic aneurysm repair was first performed by Juan Parodi in 1991 using a balloon-expandable stent to attach a Dacron polyester fabric graft to the normal infrarenal aortic neck, thus excluding blood flow from the aneurysm sac. This new and innovative approach to treat aortic aneurysms stimulated worldwide interest and led to the rapid growth and development of the field of endovascular surgery. Over the last decade, a number of endovascular devices have been developed and evaluated in clinical trials against the standard of open surgical repair. Endovascular repair has been shown to be effective in preventing aneurysm rupture with less patient morbidity and more rapid patient recovery. This minimally invasive approach has now gained acceptance as a suitable treatment strategy for selected patients with infrarenal aneurysms. There are currently three U.S. Food and Drug Administration (FDA)–approved endovascular devices available for clinical use. Several new endovascular devices are currently in clinical trials, and it is anticipated that additional and improved devices will become available in the future.

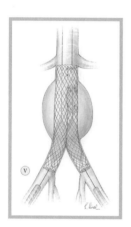

The principle of endovascular repair is similar to open surgical repair—exclusion of the aneurysm from the aortic bloodstream by attaching a prosthetic graft to the proximal nonaneurysmal aortic neck and to the iliac arteries distally. In the case of endovascular repair, attachment of the prosthetic graft is achieved by self-expanding stents that apply radial force to the normal aortic wall proximally and iliac arteries distally. A variety of endoluminal devices have been developed, including modular and unibody designs, using a variety of fixation strategies involving infrarenal and suprarenal stents, with or without hooks and barbs, combined with a varying degree of longitudinal columnar support. The technical details of deployment of each device is device specific, and each endoluminal device has its own manufacturer's specific instructions for use, which should be followed when using the device. The technique of endovascular aneurysm repair depicted in this section is based on the endoluminal device that has the largest clinical experience and longest follow-up among FDA-approved devices (AneuRx Stent Graft, Medtronic, Inc., Santa Rosa, California, FDA approved in 1999, worldwide implants >50,000).

Endovascular repair of abdominal aortic aneurysm has low perioperative morbidity and mortality rates compared with open surgery with less blood loss and transfusion requirements, shorter hospital stay, and more rapid recovery. In addition, endovascular repair may be performed in elderly, high-risk patients with multiple comorbidities who are not candidates for open surgical repair. However, not all patients with infrarenal aneurysms are candidates for endovascular repair because they do not have suitable anatomy. Whereas surgical technique may be modified and adjusted during open surgical repair to accommodate varying anatomic features of aneurysms, endovascular repair has specific morphologic requirements of the infrarenal neck and iliac arteries. Therefore, detailed preoperative imaging studies must be performed to identify patients with suitable anatomy, and an appropriately sized endoluminal device must be selected and available for successful endoluminal repair.

Preoperative examination studies include contrast CT scanning or MR angiography in patients with compromised renal function. Newer image processing techniques of 3D image reconstruction are useful to facilitate the determination of aortic neck and iliac diameter and length, particularly in patients with tortuous anatomy. These studies may be supplemented by contrast arteriography as needed. Morphologic requirements for endovascular repair using currently available devices include an infrarenal aortic neck diameter no larger than 26 mm and an aortic neck length of at least 15 mm without excessive angulation. Common iliac artery diameter should be 15 mm or less in diameter with a length of at least 20 mm. Other factors that are important in proper patient selection are aortic and iliac angulation and tortuousity, calcification and intraluminal plaque or thrombus, and iliac aneurysms and stenoses. In addition, the diameter of the common femoral and external iliac arteries should be 7 mm or greater to allow passage of large-diameter device delivery catheters. Women, in particular, often have small femoral and external iliac arteries, which often preclude transfemoral endovascular repair. In patients with small, tortuous, calcified, or severely diseased iliofemoral vessels, access technique may be modified by retroperitoneal exposure of the iliac artery and anastomosing an 8-mm Dacron polyester conduit of the external or common iliac artery to facilitate safe introduction of the endovascular device. Approximately 50% of patients with abdominal aneurysms can be treated using currently available devices. The most common morphologic feature that precludes endovascular repair is an unsuitable infrarenal aortic neck—too large, too short, or too angulated. Endovascular devices that can treat patients with larger diameter infrarenal aortic necks are currently in clinical trials, and newer juxtarenal and transrenal fixation strategies are being investigated. When such devices become available, the total number of patients who are suitable candidates for endovascular repair will increase.

The 30-day mortality rate after endovascular repair is 1% to 2% with rapid patient recovery. However, patients undergoing endovascular repair require postprocedure imaging studies to ensure that the aneurysm sac is excluded from the aortic circulation. Flow may persist in the aortic sac because of insecure fixation and seal at the aortic neck or iliac arteries (type I endoleak), insecure fixation and seal at a modular junction (type III endoleak), or retrograde flow into the aneurysm sac from lumbar arteries, the inferior mesenteric artery, or both (type II endoleak). Type I and III endoleaks require treatment to prevent subsequent aneurysm rupture. The significance of type II endoleaks is unclear, and treatment is usually required only if there is evidence of continued aneurysm enlargement.

Postprocedure follow up of patients treated with endovascular aneurysm repair includes serial follow-up imaging with contrast CT scanning, MR angiography, Duplex ultrasound and/or abdominal X-ray images to determine aneurysm size, device location and position, and the presence or absence of endoleak. Long-term problems with endografts include endoleak, aneurysm enlargement, aneurysm rupture, device migration, device disruption, graft limb thrombosis, and the need for secondary procedures, including conversion to open surgical repair. Although these problems are not common, they require close surveillance and continued monitoring of patients who undergo endovascular repair.

The patient is positioned supine on a moveable fluoroscopy table, under general or regional anesthesia. A fixed or portable C-arm image intensifier is used for intraoperative imaging. Fluoroscopic and angiographic imaging may be supplemented by intravascular ultrasound.

Small transverse incisions over the inguinal ligament (incision #l) are used to expose the common femoral arteries bilaterally. In the event the proximal common femoral artery is found to be too small or too diseased to introduce the endovascular device delivery system, the incisions may be enlarged laterally and obliquely for more proximal exposure of the external iliac or common iliac arteries. When preoperative imaging studies demonstrate small, tortuous, or diseased external iliac arteries, or when internal iliac revascularization or iliac conduits are planned, a transverse, suprainguinal incision is used (incision #2). The abdominal wall musculofascial layers are divided with retroperitoneal exposure of the external, internal, and common iliac arteries as needed. The use of a self-retaining retractor facilitates exposure.

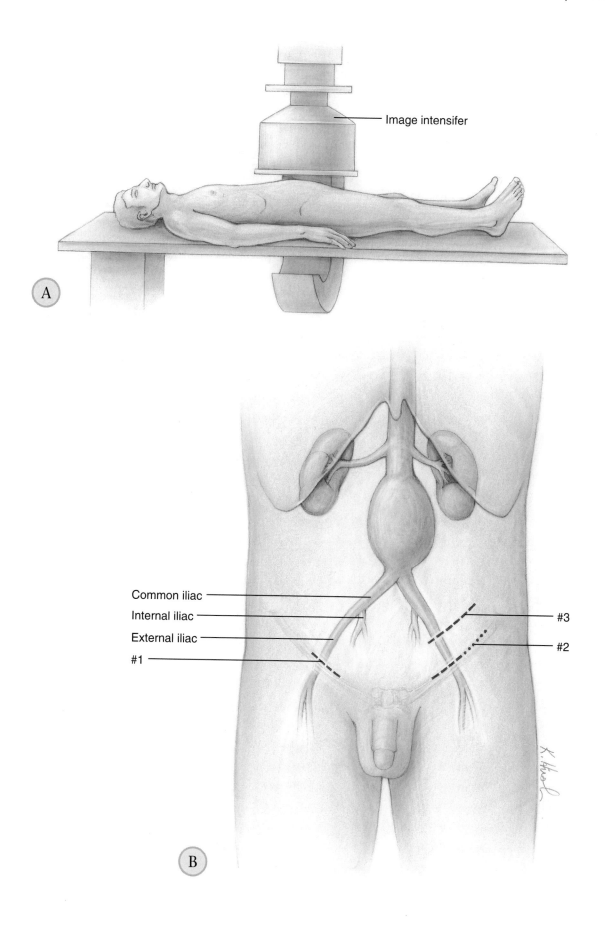

Image intensifer

Common iliac

Internal iliac

External iliac

#1

#3

#2

A

B

C The anterior wall of the common femoral artery is punctured using a Cournand needle, and a soft, flexible guidewire is introduced into the external iliac artery and advanced into the aorta. A long, 9 or 10F sheath is passed over the guidewire into the aneurysm sac. In cases of iliac tortuosity, small, short sheaths, glide wires, and glide catheters may be used to introduce a stiff wire into the supraceliac and descending thoracic aorta to facilitate introduction of the 10F sheath. This procedure is performed bilaterally. The patient is anticoagulated with systemic heparin during the procedure.

D In cases where an iliac conduit is needed because of a small or severely diseased external iliac artery, the self-retaining retractors are removed after completion of the anastomosis of the conduit to the proximal external iliac artery or common iliac artery. The 8- or 10-mm Dacron polyester conduit is brought out from the incision, clamped distally, and then punctured with a Cournand needle as in **C.** The guidewire and sheath are then introduced as described in **C.** An umbilical tape or snare is used to constrict the conduit around the sheath in the event of bleeding around the sheath.

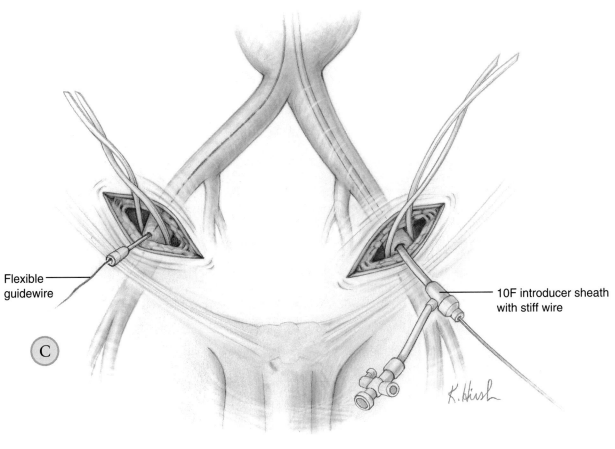

Flexible guidewire

10F introducer sheath with stiff wire

C

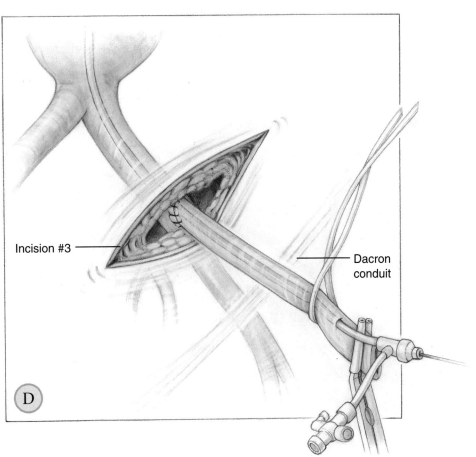

Incision #3

Dacron conduit

D

(E) A stiff guidewire is introduced into the supraceliac aorta and advanced to the descending thoracic aorta on the side that has been selected for delivery of the primary bifurcation module (right side). An angiographic catheter with sideholes for injection of contrast is introduced over a guidewire from the opposite side and positioned in the suprarenal aorta at the level of the L1 vertebral body. A pigtail or straight angiographic catheter may be used.

(F) The guidewire is withdrawn from the angiographic catheter, and an aortogram may be performed to identify the renal arteries, aneurysm, and iliac arteries. Use of an angiographic catheter with radiopaque markers at 1-cm intervals facilitates length determination and confirmation of device selection. In patients with compromised renal function and satisfactory preoperative three-dimensional imaging studies, the initial aortogram may be omitted to reduce contrast load, because the general position of the renal arteries can be localized at the top of the L2 vertebral body. The 10F sheath is removed from the right femoral artery, and the tapered nosecone of the bifurcation delivery catheter is introduced into the femoral artery over the stiff guidewire. The delivery catheter is advanced to the suprarenal aorta under fluoroscopic imaging control and rotated so that the side of the bifurcation module that has the open iliac limb faces toward the angiographic catheter, to facilitate subsequent cannulation of the iliac gate.

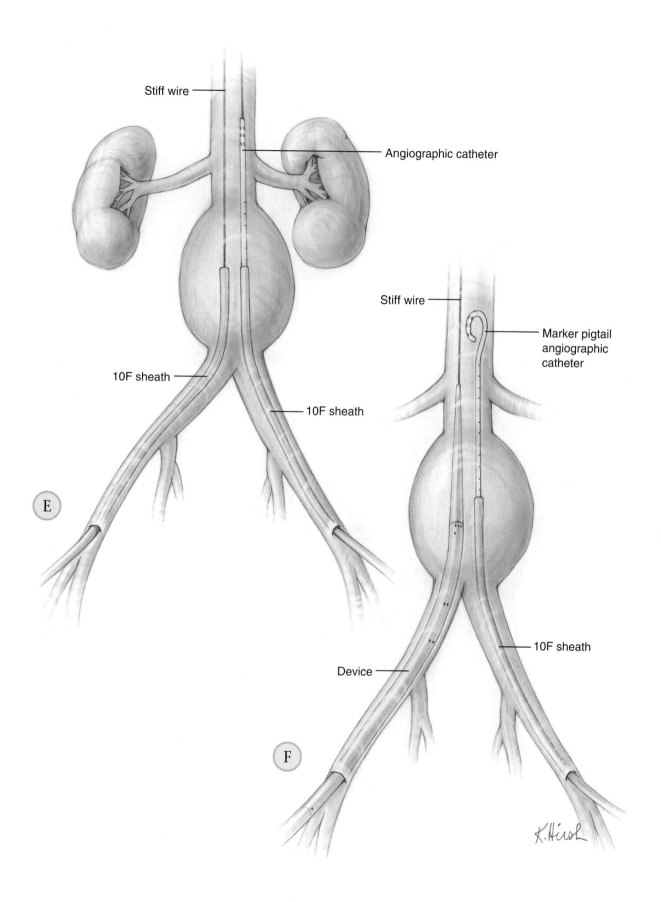

Stiff wire

Angiographic catheter

Stiff wire

Marker pigtail
angiographic
catheter

10F sheath

10F sheath

10F sheath

E

Device

F

The fluoroscopic table is then moved so that the image intensifier is positioned with the renal arteries in the center of imaging field to reduce parallax. The C-arm gantry is angulated cranially and rotated to the side as needed to optimally image the renal arteries and infrarenal aortic neck, on the basis of preoperative three-dimensional imaging studies. A magnified image aortogram is then obtained to precisely localize the renal arteries. The top of the stent graft is positioned just above the renal arteries. When proper positioning is obtained, the table and imager are locked into place.

The covering sheath of the delivery catheter is then retracted using the deployment handle. This exposes the top of the self-expanding stent graft. The delivery system is slowly withdrawn as the stent graft begins to expand to a position immediately below the lowermost renal artery.

The stent graft is withdrawn so that the top of the stent graft is just below the lowermost renal artery. Repeated angiographic "puffs" can be performed through the angiographic catheter to reconfirm the position of the top of the stent graft in relation to the renal arteries. The covering sheath is slowly retracted allowing the stent graft to expand and apply radial fixation force to the infrarenal aortic neck. Note that the angiographic catheter is outside of the stent graft, between the stent graft and the aortic wall. The catheter stays in this position until the covering sheath is fully retracted allowing fixation both proximally in the infrarenal aortic neck and distally in the iliac artery. A guidewire is then introduced into the angiographic catheter to straighten the pigtail, and the catheter is withdrawn into the aneurysm sac. This catheter will then be replaced by an angled catheter to allow introduction of the guidewire and catheter into the open iliac limb and through the lumen of the stent graft to the suprarenal aorta.

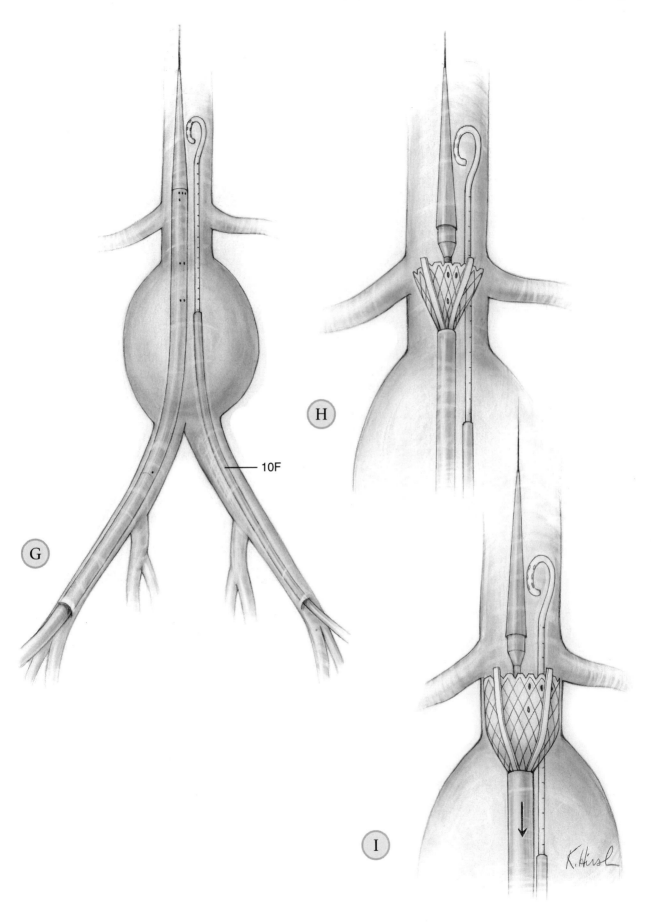

10F

G

H

I

The primary bifurcation module is fully expanded. The tapered introducer nosecone and metallic "runners" that are on the outside of the stent graft are shown. The metallic runners separate the stent graft from the covering sheath and reduce friction during sheath retraction. The nosecone and runners may now be retracted, leaving the stiff guidewire in place within the fully deployed bifurcation module (see panel **K**). Alternatively, the nosecone and runners may be left in place at this point and retracted after deployment of the contralateral iliac limb (see panels **Q–S**). This minimizes the potential risk for movement of the bifurcation module during retraction of the runners and is particularly useful when treating patients with short, angulated aortic necks.

A guidewire is then introduced into the open iliac gate of the stent graft within the aneurysm sac. Cannulation of the open gate is facilitated by using an angled glide wire and an angled catheter with rotation of the C-arm gantry side-to-side to best visualize the open gate. Differing shaped and angled catheters may be needed for retrograde cannulation in some patients with severe angulations and tortuosities. If retrograde cannulation is not successful, one may snare the guidewire from the opposite side (see panel **P**). It is important to confirm that the guidewire and catheter is through the open gate and not behind or in front of it by rotation of the C-arm side-to-side. Correct cannulation of the iliac gate can also be confirmed by intravascular ultrasound or rotation of a reformed pigtail catheter within the stent graft.

The primary module has been deployed, and the nosecone and "runners" have been retracted, leaving a stiff guidewire in place on the right side. The delivery catheter is removed from the right side and replaced with a 16F sheath, to provide hemostasis and a working port. A guidewire and catheter have been introduced into the opposite open iliac gate, and the soft glide wire has been replaced by a stiff guidewire. An angiographic catheter with 1-cm markers has been placed on the stiff guidewire. The 10F sheath is then withdrawn to the left external iliac artery, and a retrograde arteriogram is performed through the sheath to identify the position of the hypogastric artery. This allows measurement of iliac length from the top of the junction gate to the hypogastric orifice. The optimum length iliac limb can thus be selected, and a decision can be made regarding the need for an iliac extender cuff. It is desirable to obtain the maximum possible iliac fixation length without obstructing the hypogastric artery. Similar retrograde iliac arteriography can then be performed on the left side to determine the distance from the end of the primary module to the right hypogastric artery and to determine if an extender cuff is needed on that side.

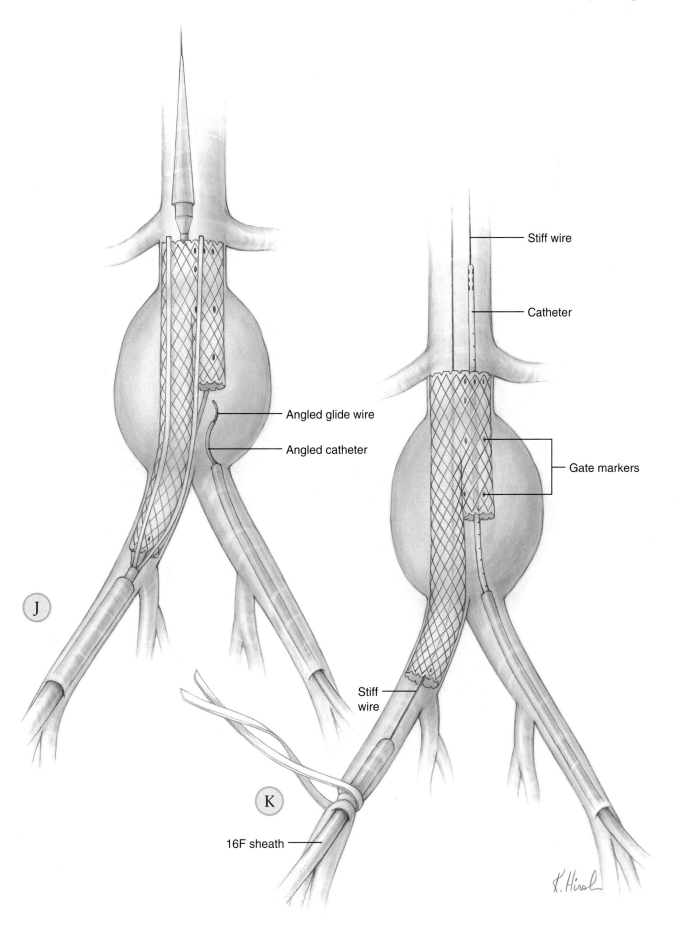

Stiff wire

Catheter

Angled glide wire

Angled catheter

Gate markers

Stiff wire

J

K

16F sheath

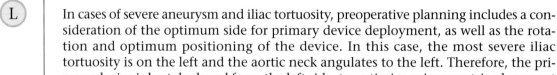

L In cases of severe aneurysm and iliac tortuosity, preoperative planning includes a consideration of the optimum side for primary device deployment, as well as the rotation and optimum positioning of the device. In this case, the most severe iliac tortuosity is on the left and the aortic neck angulates to the left. Therefore, the primary device is best deployed from the left side, to optimize axisymmetric placement of the proximal portion of the stent graft below the renal arteries. The severe tortuosity will be largely straightened by the stiff guidewire and cannulation of the open gate will be easier from the less tortuous side.

M The guidewires and catheters from the right and left sides cross within the aneurysm sac because of the angulation and tortuosity of the iliac arteries. In this circumstance, the primary bifurcation module, coming from the left side, should be rotated so that the open gate is to the left, where the guidewire from the right femoral artery is located.

N After deployment of the bifurcation module, the open iliac limb is on the left side, thus facilitating cannulation of the open gate by the guidewire from the right groin. Rotation of the bifurcation module in this manner increases the length requirement of the iliac limb to reach the iliac artery. Length measurement should be made and an iliac extender limb should be placed, if necessary, to achieve at least 3 cm of iliac fixation length.

O The two limbs of the bifurcation graft are crossed. This position results in less severe angulation of each iliac limb and reduces the risk for kinking and angulation of the limbs of the stent graft.

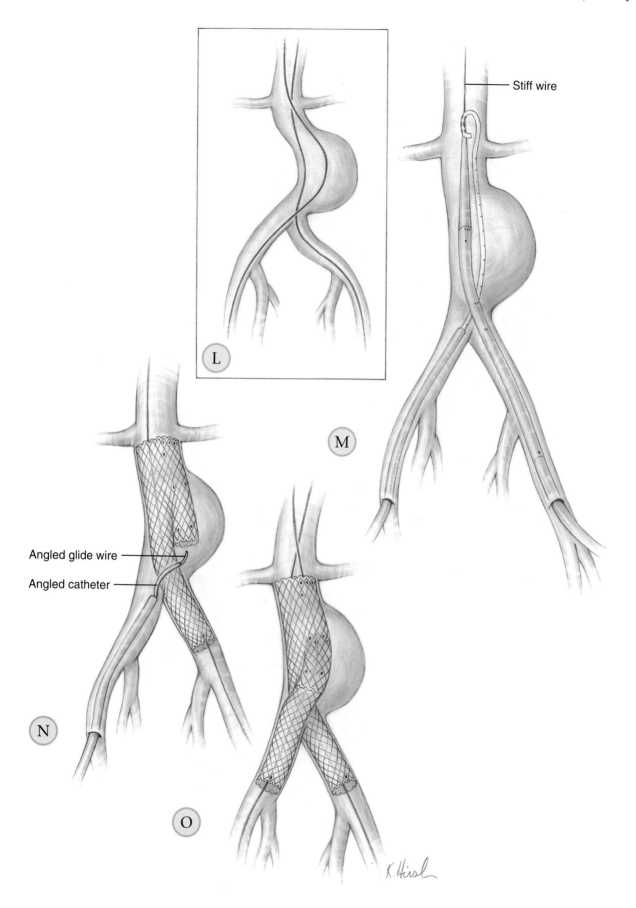

Cannulation of open iliac gate using a crosswire and snare. A shepherd's crook catheter is passed over a guidewire from the right groin and reformed in the supraceliac aorta. The shepherd's crook is brought down into the stent graft and positioned in the open left iliac limb. An angled glide wire is passed from the right groin, over the bifurcation, and down into the aneurysm sac where it is snared by a wire from the left groin. The wire is extracted from the left groin and used to pass a catheter through the open gate and into the aorta. This catheter is then used to introduce a stiff wire from the left groin through the open iliac limb.

The 10F sheath is removed from the left groin, and the iliac limb delivery catheter is passed over the stiff wire and through the iliac junction gate. The iliac junction gate is 2.5 cm in length and is marked by four radiopaque markers, two proximal and two distal. The distal end of the stent graft is visible, and note of its relation to the hypogastric artery should be made. The iliac limb has radiopaque markers proximally and distally.

The image intensifier is positioned over the iliac junction gate, and magnification is used as necessary for optimal visualization of the gate markers. The proximal iliac limb marker must be positioned within the 2.5-cm-long marker gate. In cases where there is significant tortuosity and iliac angulation, the iliac limb marker should be placed near the top of the gate to maximize device overlap. The covering sheath of the delivery catheter is retracted using the deployment handle, thus allowing the self-expanding iliac stent graft module to expand. Radial expansion force of the iliac stent fixes the module in place in the junction gate.

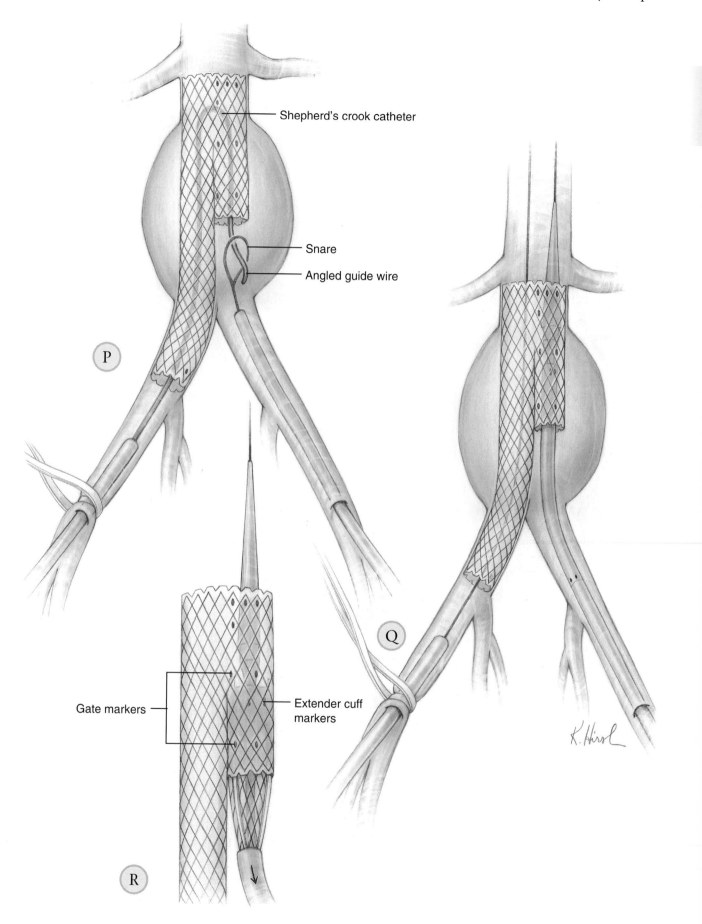

Shepherd's crook catheter

Snare

Angled guide wire

P

Q

Gate markers

Extender cuff markers

R

K. Hirsl

The left iliac limb is fully expanded, and the nosecone and "runners" of the delivery catheter have been retracted and removed. The bifurcated stent graft is now fully deployed. The stiff guidewire is left in place. A 16F sheath is placed in the left femoral artery to provide hemostasis and a working port. A pigtail catheter may be introduced into the proximal aorta for a completion aortogram. Particular attention is paid to the proximal and distal fixation zones to ensure that there is no type I endoleak. Retrograde iliac angiograms may be performed to identify the hypogastric arteries and to better define the distal fixation zone. Iliac extender modules are used if iliac fixation length is less than 3 cm and may be used to extend the stent graft to the level of the internal iliac arteries.

A left iliac extender module has been deployed to extend the stent graft to the level of the left internal iliac artery. A right iliac extender module delivery catheter is in place, ready for device deployment. The use of proximal and distal extender modules increases device fixation length and reduces the possibility of device migration.

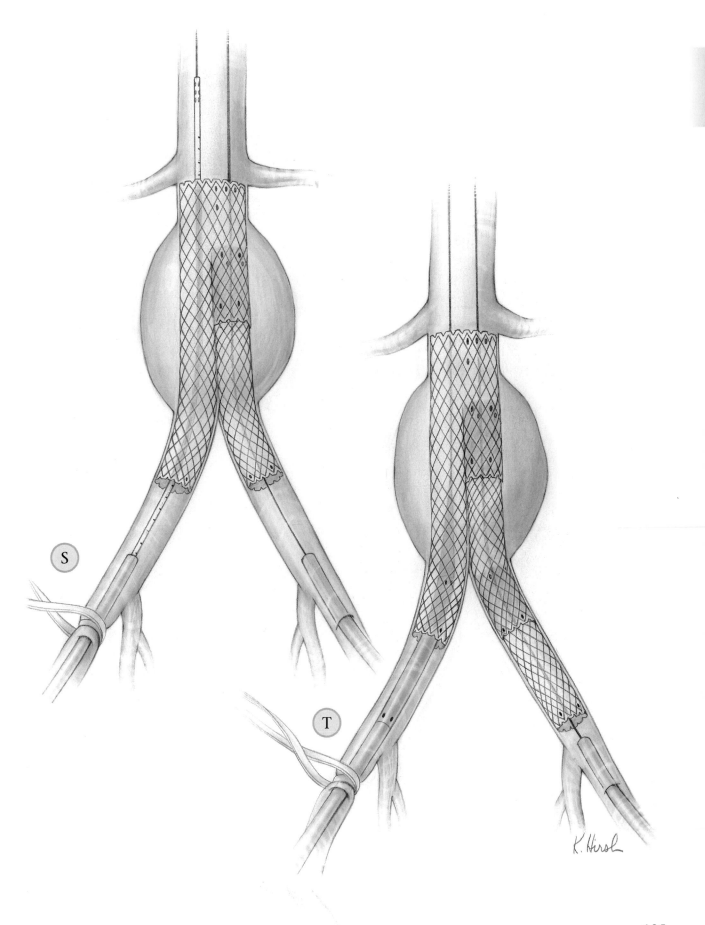

Small or normal caliber distal aortas and stenotic iliac segments should be balloon dilated to fully expand the stent graft. Appropriately sized noncompliant balloons are used in the iliac limbs, and a low-pressure compliant aortic balloon may be used proximally.

Bilateral noncompliant balloons are introduced over the guidewires and inflated within the stent graft at 4 to 5 atm using the "kissing balloon" technique. Care must be taken so that the shoulders of the balloons do not extend outside of the stent graft to avoid iliac artery rupture.

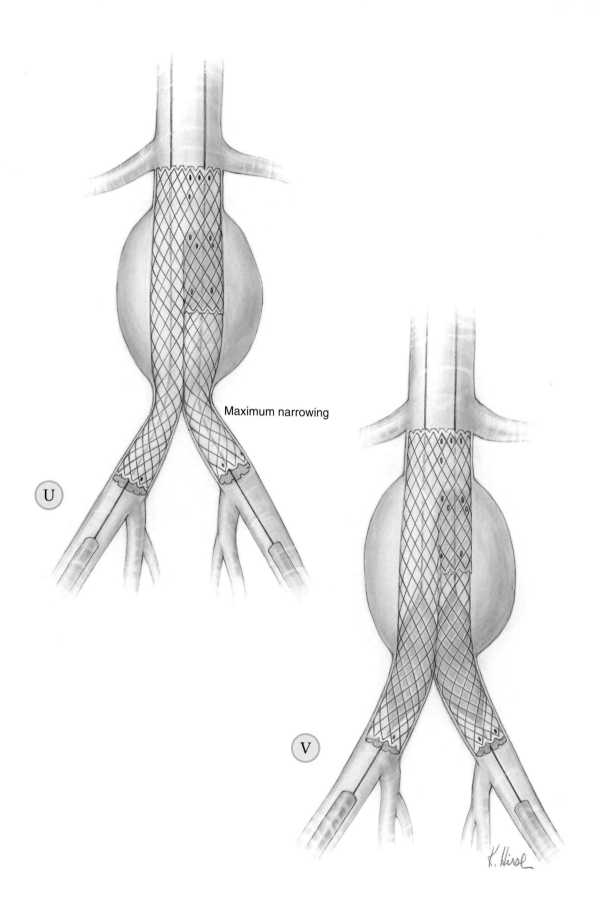

Maximum narrowing

U

V

K. Hirsl

Coil Embolization of Internal Iliac Artery

Internal iliac (hypogastric) aneurysms may be excluded from the circulation by coil embolization of the distal branches of the hypogastric artery and extending the stent graft into the external iliac artery.

A guidewire is passed across the iliac bifurcation and directed into the distal branches of the internal iliac artery past the aneurysm. A catheter is introduced over the guidewire into the branch vessel and is used to deliver coils into the distal branch vessels. Each branch of the internal iliac artery is catheterized and multiple coils are needed to occlude each branch in order to prevent retrograde filling of the aneurysm. A guiding sheath is used over the iliac bifurcation to facilitate catheter and guidewire manipulation.

After coiling of the distal branches, an iliac extender module is used to cover the orifice of the internal iliac artery and to exclude the aneurysm from the circulation. The iliac extender module should extend at least 2.5 cm into the external iliac artery.

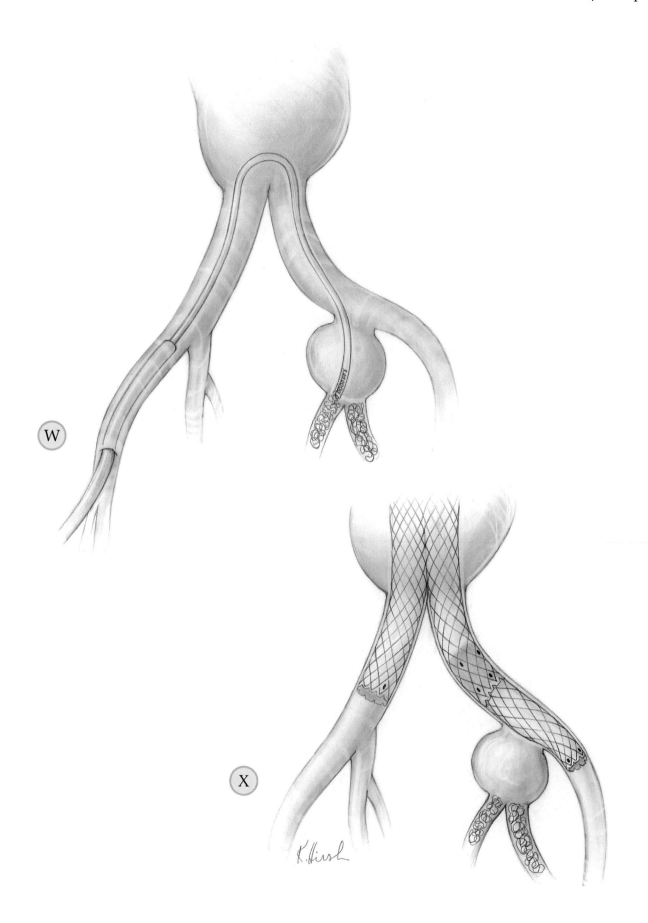

Preservation of the Internal Iliac Artery

Common iliac aneurysm, which extends to the level of the iliac bifurcation, provides no suitable fixation zone in the common iliac artery.

The iliac bifurcation is exposed through a retroperitoneal approach, and the internal iliac artery is mobilized, clamped, and transected. The proximal stump is oversewn with 4–0 polypropylene suture. A 6-mm Dacron graft is sutured end-to-end to the distal internal iliac artery using 5–0 polypropylene suture. The bypass graft to the distal internal iliac artery is clamped for later anastomosis to the external iliac artery (see Fig. D). A guidewire and sheath are then introduced into the external iliac artery and the stent graft is deployed as previously described.

An 8-mm conduit may be anastomosed to the external iliac artery to facilitate introduction of the stent graft and then anastomosed to the internal iliac bypass graft at the completion of the stent graft procedure.

Iliac extender modules are used to extend the stent graft into the external iliac artery. This completely excludes the common iliac aneurysm and covers the orifice of the internal iliac artery. The hypogastric bypass is anastomosed to the external iliac artery using 5–0 polypropylene suture.

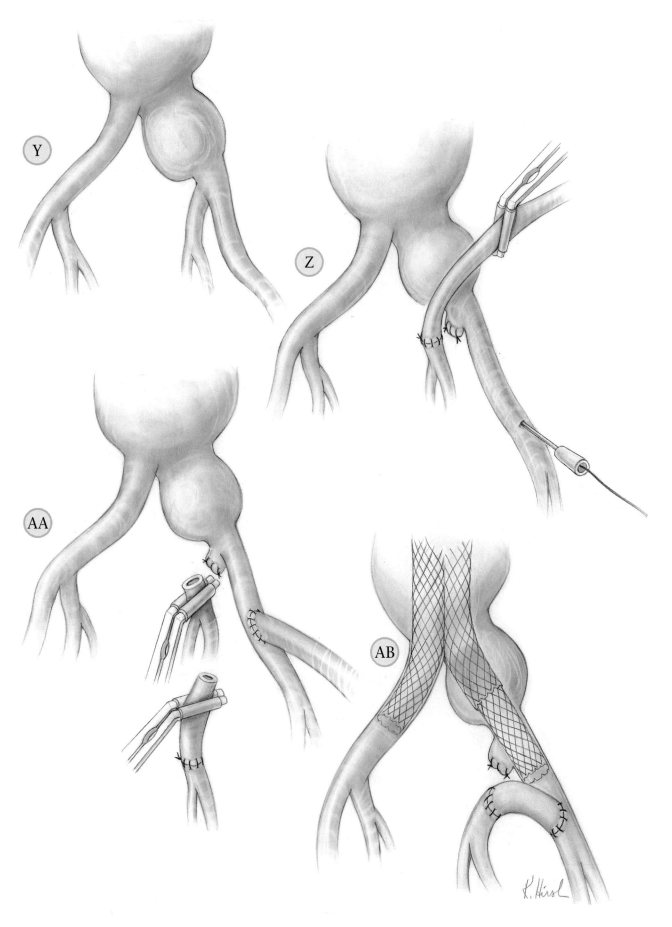

Iliac and Femoral Artery Closure

After endovascular device deployment and completion arteriography, the guidewires and sheaths are removed and the access arteriotomies are closed. Several methods of closure are available, such as those shown in panels **A** through **F.**

After endovascular device deployment and completion arteriography, retractors are positioned to expose the femoral artery in the groin. A vascular clamp is placed on the distal common femoral artery before removal of the sheath to prevent dislodgement of plaque or thrombus into the distal femoral artery. The sheath and guidewire are then removed, the proximal artery is flushed, and a proximal clamp is placed on the common femoral artery.

The femoral artery is inspected and most often can be repaired primarily with interrupted 5–0 monofilament sutures.

In the event of irregular plaque or intimal flap, the arteriotomy incision may be extended longitudinally and the artery may be repaired with a patch angioplasty, with or without endarterectomy.

In the event of extensive disruption of the femoral artery or plaque, the artery may be repaired with a local interposition graft using 6- or 8-m prosthetic graft material.

After device deployment through an iliac access conduit, the guidewire and sheath are removed and the conduit is flushed and then clamped close to the anastomosis. There is usually no need to reclamp the iliac artery. The conduit may be oversewn leaving a short stump that acts as a patch angioplasty.

In the event of severe external iliac occlusive disease, tortuosity, or dissection, the distal end of the iliac access conduit may be anastomosed to the common femoral artery in an end-to-side or end-to-end fashion. This results in an iliofemoral bypass reconstruction or iliofemoral interposition graft reconstruction.

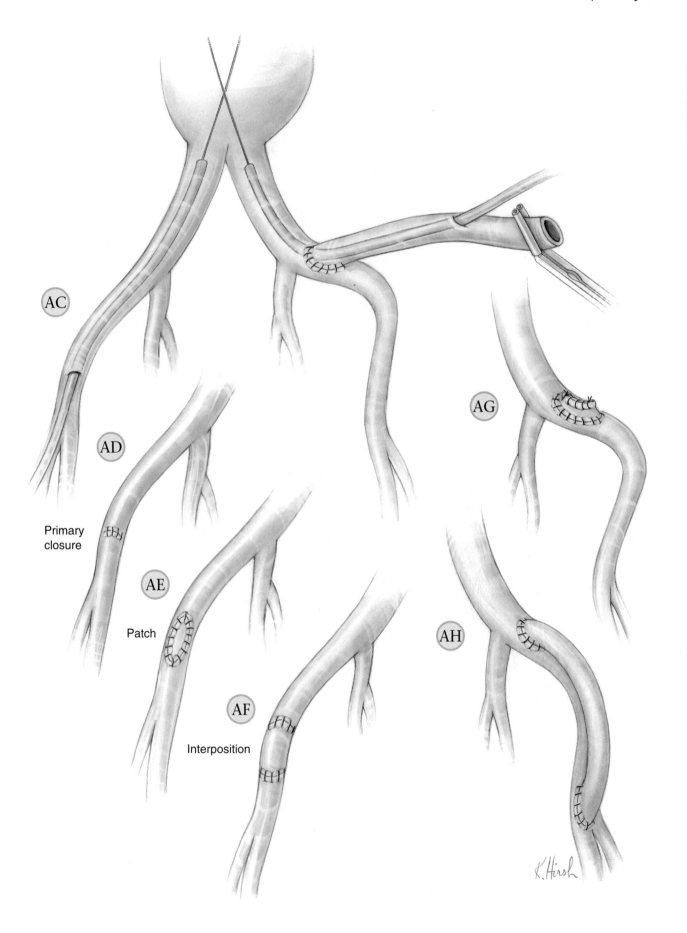

AC

AD

Primary
closure

AE

Patch

AF

Interposition

AG

AH

K. Hirsh

The natural history of ruptured abdominal aortic aneurysms is exsanguinating hemorrhage and death. More than 50% of patients who sustain aneurysm rupture will die before receiving medical attention. Among those with contained rupture who survive and reach a hospital, less than half survive emergency surgery.

Patients with ruptured abdominal aortic aneurysms should have placement of large-bore central venous catheters for fluid resuscitation and should be transported immediately to the operating room. Other diagnostic tests for patients in shock are not necessary and serve only to delay the essential surgical care.

The patient is positioned on the operating table, and the abdomen is prepared and draped with the patient awake so that immediate laparotomy can be performed should hypotension develop on induction of general anesthesia. Anesthetic agents commonly cause peripheral vasodilation and may result in sudden hypotension in marginally compensated patients.

The primary and most immediate objective in emergent repair of ruptured abdominal aortic aneurysms is to obtain rapid control of the aorta proximal to the ruptured aneurysm to prevent exsanguinating hemorrhage. This can be accomplished by transabdominal exposure of the supraceliac aorta at the aortic hiatus of the diaphragm with manual compression of the aorta against the spine or, preferably, separation or division of the fibers of the left crus of the diaphragm to expose the supraceliac aorta so that an aortic cross clamp can be applied. This maneuver avoids opening the retroperitoneum over the ruptured aneurysm and exacerbating hemorrhage that may have been tamponaded. After the supraceliac aorta is cross-clamped, the hematoma is opened and the infrarenal aortic neck is identified and controlled below the renal arteries. An infrarenal aortic cross clamp can then be applied and the supraceliac clamp released. Extensive dissection of the iliac arteries is usually not necessary to obtain distal control and should be avoided to reduce the risk for iliac vein injury. If clamps cannot be readily applied to the iliac arteries, balloon occlusion of the iliac arteries from within the aneurysm may be considered. After vascular control is obtained, a tube or bifurcated Dacron polyester graft is sutured in place to restore flow in the aorta.

Alternate methods of emergent aortic control include balloon occlusion of the proximal aorta. Although some investigators have recommended introducing the aortic occlusion balloon from within the ruptured aneurysm, this method usually is associated with extensive blood loss and may be ineffective. The availability of C-arm fluoroscopic imaging in the operating room allows the introduction of an aortic occlusion balloon over a transfemoral or transbrachial guidewire and precise positioning of the balloon in the aorta proximal to the rupture. This technique of endovascular control and aortic occlusion minimizes the risk for shock and cardiac arrest on opening the abdomen in patients with extensive intraabdominal hemorrhage and abdominal tamponade. Restricted fluid resuscitation and tolerance of low blood pressure during transport to the operating room can reduce the risk for aortic bleeding during preparation for surgery and allow time for angiography in the operating room, placement of guidewires, and proper positioning of occlusion balloons in the aorta. The aortic occlusion balloons can then be inflated as needed during operative repair of the aneurysm.

Emergent operating room angiographic evaluation of patients with rupture can also identify patients who may be candidates for endovascular treatment of the ruptured aneurysm. Currently, almost 400 patients with ruptured abdominal aortic aneurysms have been treated with aortic endografts worldwide. Favorable early results have been reported from several centers with operative mortality rates of 10% to 45% in high-risk patients. However, the number of patients treated to date is small, and the role of endovascular techniques in the treatment of patients with ruptured abdominal aortic aneurysms remains unclear. It is likely that this approach will gain wider acceptance in the future as endovascular technology continues to improve.

Patients with ruptured abdominal aortic aneurysms usually present with the sudden onset of back or abdominal pain and hypotension. Many patients have pulsatile abdominal masses, although this may not always be apparent in obese patients.

The abdomen is entered through a long midline incision extending from the xiphoid process to the pubis. The location and extent of the retroperitoneal hematoma and the size of the aneurysm determine whether initial control of the aorta will be obtained below the renal arteries or at the level of the diaphragm. If the hematoma has not obscured and distorted the location of the duodenum and left renal vein, initial control is obtained below the level of the renal arteries. The peritoneum overlying the hematoma and aneurysm is incised to the left of the duodenum, and the infrarenal aorta is isolated by blunt finger dissection through the hematoma. Care must be exercised to avoid injury to the duodenum. Dissection is minimal and is limited to what is required to clamp the infrarenal aorta.

The infrarenal aorta is cross-clamped with a long straight or curved vascular clamp below the level of the renal arteries. Systemic heparinization is usually not used in patients with ruptured abdominal aneurysms. It should be recognized, however, that distal intravascular thrombosis can develop. Regional heparinization through direct injection into the iliac arteries can minimize this possibility.

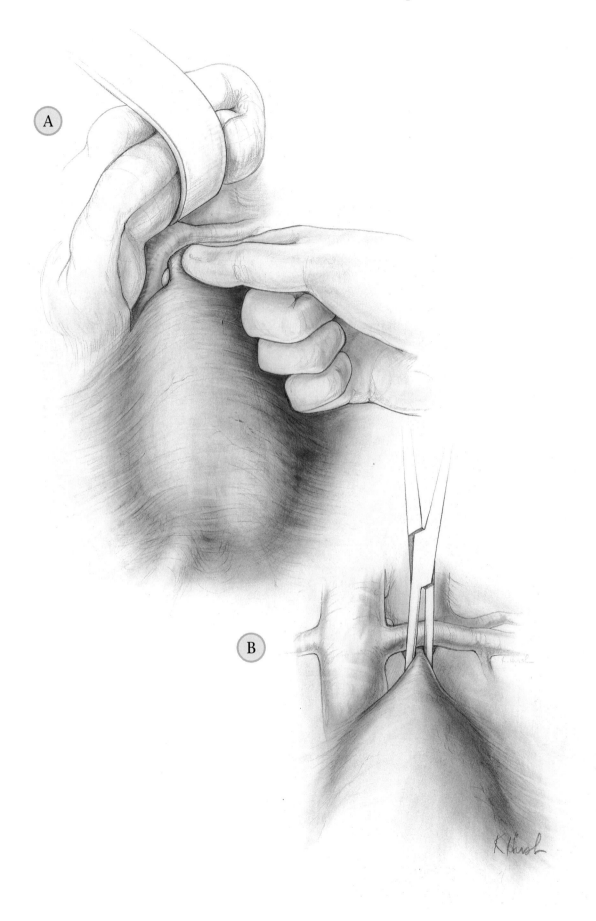

An alternative means of obtaining rapid proximal aortic control is to inflate a large balloon catheter in the suprarenal aorta. This catheter is best passed through an incision in the anterior wall of the aneurysm. After inflation of the balloon, the neck of the aneurysm is exposed below the level of the renal arteries, the balloon catheter is removed and the infrarenal aorta cross-clamped.

In patients with a large retroperitoneal hematoma extending above the level of the renal vein, it is usually best to occlude the aorta at the level of the diaphragm. The lesser curvature of the stomach is retracted inferiorly, and the supraceliac aorta is identified as it passes through the diaphragmatic crura behind and to the right of the esophagus. The aorta can be cross-clamped at this level with a long curved or straight vascular clamp or occluded by compressing the aorta against the underlying vertebral bodies using a sponge stick (as shown). The retroperitoneum over the aneurysm is then incised and the infrarenal aorta is isolated using blunt dissection within the hematoma. After infrarenal control is obtained, supraceliac aortic occlusion is released.

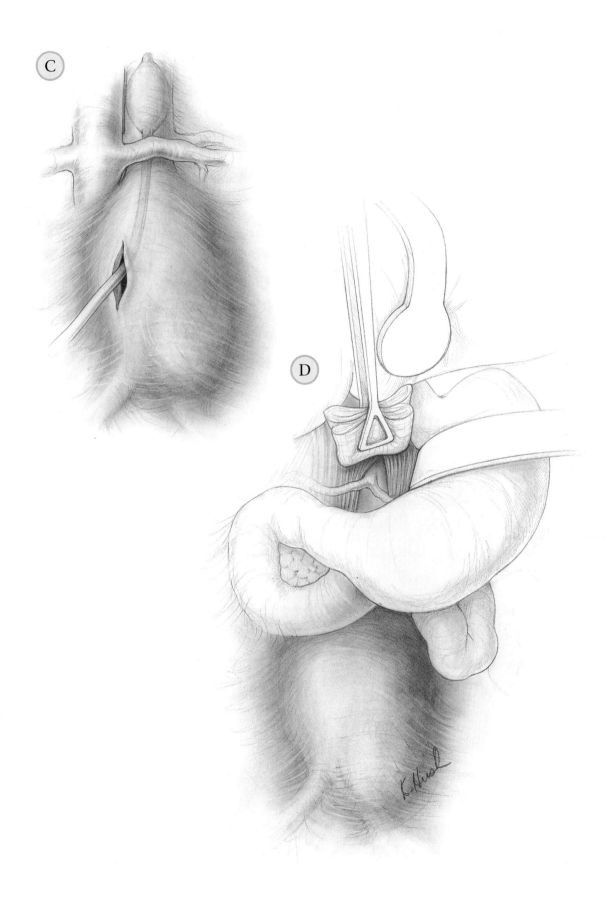

If the iliac arteries are easily identified, they should be clamped after minimal dissection as shown on page 67. In the presence of an extensive hematoma obscuring the iliac vessels, distal vascular control may be obtained by intraluminal balloon tamponade after opening the aneurysm widely. Mural thrombus is removed and lumbar and inferior mesenteric artery back bleeding is controlled by suture ligation from within the aneurysm. A tightly woven rather than knitted Dacron graft should be used to minimize blood loss through the interstices of the graft. The graft is sutured within the aneurysm using large and deep continuous sutures (see page 65).

A tube graft aortic reconstruction is most commonly used for ruptured aortic aneurysm repair. However, if the iliac arteries are aneurysmal, an aortoiliac bypass may be necessary. Before completion of the distal anastomosis, patency of the iliac arteries must be ascertained to rule out the possibility of distal thrombus formation during the initial aortic occlusion without heparin. The iliac occluding balloon catheters are deflated and back bleeding is assessed. If no back bleeding is obtained, embolectomy catheters should be passed down the iliac arteries and thrombus should be extracted. The iliac balloon catheters are deflated and withdrawn through the suture line just before suture completion at the distal aorta. The aneurysm wall is then closed over the graft and the retroperitoneum is closed as shown on page 67.

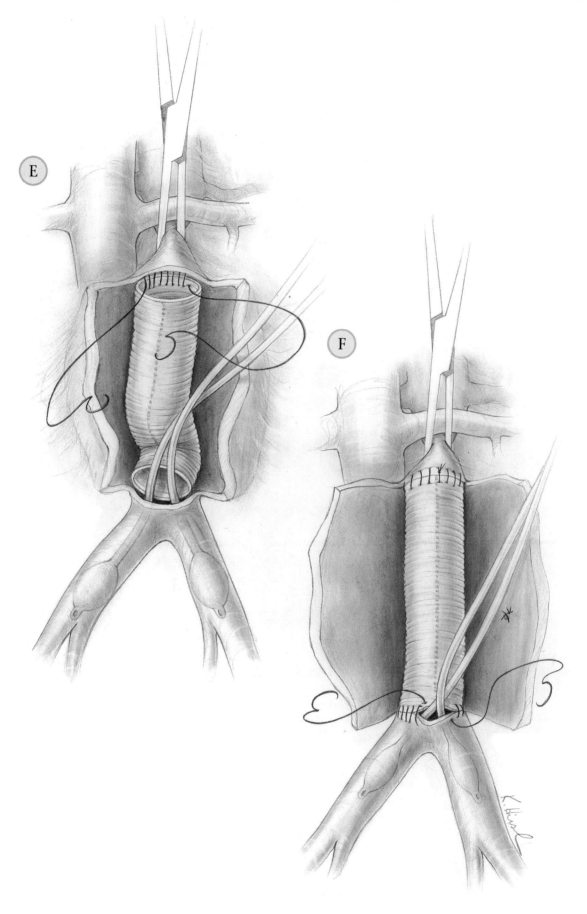

Thoracoabdominal aortic aneurysms involve all or part of the descending thoracic aorta, as well as all or part of the abdominal aorta and iliac arteries. Stanley Crawford's classification of thoracoabdominal aneurysms is based on the pattern and extent of the aneurysm. Type I thoracoabdominal aneurysms involve all or most of the descending thoracic aorta and the upper abdominal aorta, ending above the renal arteries. Type II aneurysms have similar involvement of the descending thoracic aorta as Type I, but extend to involve the abdominal aorta below the renal arteries. Type III aneurysms involve the distal half of the descending thoracic aorta together with varying involvement of the abdominal aorta. Type IV thoracoabdominal aneurysms begin at or just above the diaphragm and include all or most of the segment of abdominal aorta from which the visceral vessels arise. The most common cause of thoracoabdominal aortic aneurysm is atherosclerotic aortic wall degeneration (82%), followed by aortic dissection (17%). Uncommon etiologic factors include mycotic aneurysm, Takayasu arteritis, Marfan's syndrome, and Ehlers-Danlos syndrome. More than 40% of patients with atherosclerotic aneurysms are asymptomatic at the time of diagnosis compared with only 15% of patients with aortic dissections. The most common symptom in both types of aortic degeneration is pain. Pain can be acute or insidious and can appear in the chest, back, flank, or abdomen. More uncommon symptoms include wheezing, hoarseness, dyspnea, recurrent pulmonary infections, dysphagia, ureteral obstruction, and small bowel ischemia. Acute aortic dissection can cause renal ischemia (12%), visceral ischemia (9%), acute leg ischemia (9%), and paraplegia or paraparesis (3%).

The risk for rupture of thoracoabdominal aortic aneurysms is high, with rupture and death occurring in 40% to 70% of patients with untreated thoracic and thoracoabdominal aortic aneurysms. The actuarial 5-year survival rate of patients with untreated thoracic aortic aneurysm is 9% to 13%, with patients most often dying of aneurysm rupture. The most important factor predictive of rupture is aneurysm size. The maximum diameter of the descending thoracic aorta and abdominal aorta correlate best to the probability of rupture. Other factors that significantly increase the risk for rupture are advanced age, COPD, and presence of pain. Chronic renal failure has also been found to be an independent risk factor for rupture. Dr. Randall Griepp and his colleagues in New York have studied the factors predictive of rupture in untreated aneurysms and developed an equation to calculate the yearly rate of rupture (λ) according to age, maximal diameter of thoracic and abdominal aorta, and the presence or absence of pain or COPD. Using the equation $\lambda = -21.055 + 0.093(\text{age}) + 0.842(\text{pain}) + 1.282(\text{COPD}) + 0.643(\text{maximal descending thoracic diameter}) + 0.405(\text{maximal abdominal aortic diameter})$, the 1-year risk for rupture in a 65-year-old patient with a thoracoabdominal aortic aneurysm (5 cm in abdominal aorta and 6 cm in thoracic aorta) without pain or COPD is 4%. The 1-year risk for rupture in a thoracobadominal aneurysm of the same dimensions in a 75-year-old patient with COPD or with COPD and pain is 30% and 56%, respectively.

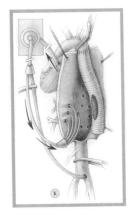

The risk for rupture of an untreated thoracoabdominal aneurysm must be weighed against the risks involved with open surgical repair. Operative repair is the recommended treatment for patients with aneurysms larger than 6 cm in diameter, provided they are suitable surgical candidates. Surgical repair requires a thoracoabdominal exposure of the aorta, tube graft replacement, and revascularization of the celiac, superior mesenteric, and both renal arteries, with or without revascularization of intercostal arteries. This may be performed with or without shunt bypass to maintain distal perfusion. The mortality rate associated with surgical repair of thoracoabdominal aneurysms is 10% to 20% and ranges from 4% to 40% depending on symptomatology and extent of the aneurysm, urgency of the procedure, and patient risk factors and comorbid conditions. Major morbidity after the procedure may include cardiac, pulmonary, renal, and multisystem organ failure, as well as paraplegia caused by spinal cord ischemia.

Type IV thoracoabdominal aneurysms begin at or just above the level of the diaphragm and involve the segment of abdominal aorta from which the visceral vessels arise. These aneurysms may be treated using an abdominal approach, thus avoiding a thoracoabdominal incision and reducing pulmonary complications and improving overall results. The aneurysm is exposed through a left flank incision and retroperitoneal approach. The peritoneum is mobilized from the diaphragm, and the left crus of the diaphragm is divided to enlarge the aortic hiatus. This provides exposure to the distal descending thoracic aorta in the posterior mediastinum for proximal aortic control. By avoiding thoracotomy and division of the diaphragm, patients recover more rapidly and have fewer perioperative complications.

Endoluminal devices have been developed for repair of thoracic aortic aneurysms and are currently undergoing U.S. clinical trials for FDA approval. Endoluminal devices for thoracic aneurysm repair are available in Europe and Australia. Early results of endovascular thoracic aortic aneurysm repair are good and the risk/benefit ratio of endoluminal repair compared with open surgical repair of thoracic aneurysms is favorable. It is anticipated that endoluminal devices for the treatment of thoracic aortic aneurysms will soon be approved by the FDA for use in the United States. Active investigation is underway to develop branched vessel endoluminal devices that can be used to treat thoracoabdominal aneurysms involving the visceral vessels.

The principles involved in the repair of thoracoabdominal aneurysm are the same as for the repair of other aneurysms in the vascular tree, namely exclusion of the aneurysm from the circulation system using a prosthetic graft while preserving vital organ blood flow. For a thoracoabdominal aneurysm this involves opening the aneurysm and placing a prosthetic graft within (endoaneurysmorrhaphy technique). Flow to the celiac, superior mesenteric, and renal arteries is provided by suturing the orifices of these vessels to an opening in the side of the graft. Maintenance of spinal cord blood flow poses a particular problem because the anterior spinal artery frequently arises from intercostal arteries exiting from the aneurysm. The risk for paraplegia with repair of extensive thoracoabdominal aneurysms is 10% to 15% even with specific measures taken to preserve or restore spinal cord blood flow. It remains uncertain whether reattachment of large intercostal and lumbar arteries to the graft decreases the risk for paraplegia. Preoperative evaluation includes aortography and computed tomography scanning to evaluate the extent of the aneurysm and visceral branches, as well as to identify large intercostal and lumbar arteries.

Anesthesia is induced with agents least likely to result in cardiac depression. A double lumen endotracheal tube is inserted so that the left lung can be deflated during exposure of the aorta. Hemodynamic monitoring is essential with radial artery and central venous pressure catheters and thermodilution catheters for delineation of cardiac output; cardiac monitoring may be further improved by transesophageal echocardiography. Multiple large-bore peripheral intravenous catheters are placed for rapid volume replacement. Mannitol is administered to promote vigorous diuresis. Proximal blood pressure, cardiac hemodynamics, and peripheral vascular resistance are maintained at desirable levels during the period of aortic clamping by the administration of vasodilators and judicious fluid replacement.

In those patients with higher cardiac risk factors or anticipated lengthy aortic clamp times (longer than 45 minutes), some form of left ventricular "unloading" may be desirable. Atrialfemoral extracorporeal bypass can be instituted both to perfuse the lower extremities and reduce ventricular afterload. As described by Safi and colleagues in Houston, Texas, this technology allows for perfusion "side arms" to cannulate the visceral vessels during aortic clamping.

The patient is positioned on the right side and held at a 60-degree angle using a bean bag. Operative exposure is obtained through an incision made in both the thoracic and abdominal cavities. The exact level is determined by the location and extent of the aneurysm. Midaortic lesions can be exposed through a ninth intercostal incision that extends obliquely across the abdomen to the midline at the level of the umbilicus. More extensive aneurysms involving most of the thoracic and abdominal aorta are best exposed through a sixth or seventh intercostal space incision crossing the costal cartilages to the midline of the abdomen and extending to the pubis.

The diaphragm may be cut radially to the aortic hiatus or circumferentially; the latter better preserves diaphragmatic innervation. The left lung is collapsed and gently retracted medially exposing the posterior mediastinum.

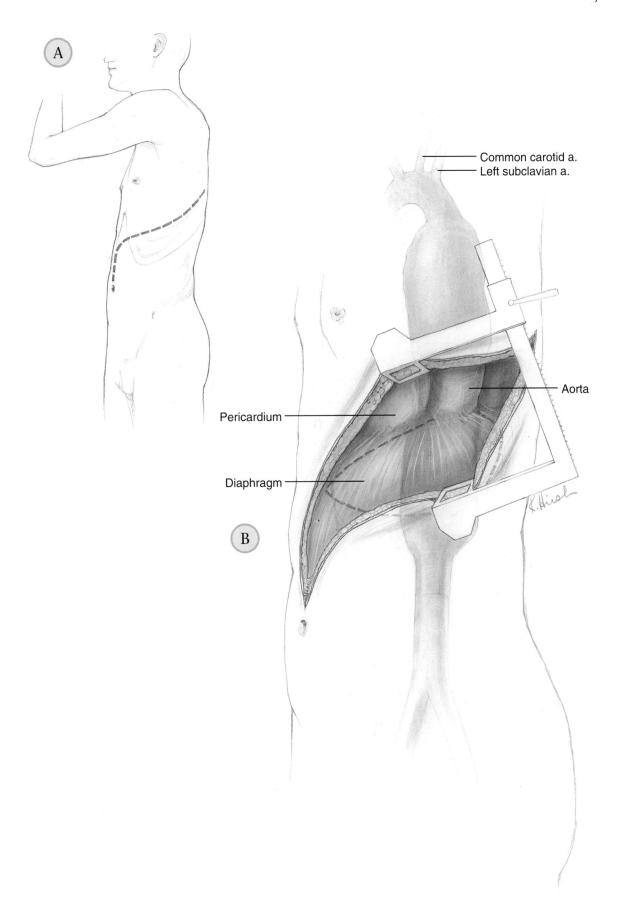

The mediastinal pleural is incised over the aorta proximal to the aneurysm. Aortic dissection in the chest is limited to mobilization of enough uninvolved proximal aorta to apply a clamp. This is accomplished by blunt digital dissection, avoiding injury to the esophagus and intercostal arteries. The abdominal aortic segment is exposed extraperitoneally, incising the peritoneum lateral to the left colon and entering the retroperitoneal space. The left colon, kidney, spleen, body and tail of the pancreas, and fundus of the stomach are mobilized and retracted to the right; this exposes the entire length of the aorta from the diaphragm to the aortic bifurcation. The abdominal aorta below the aneurysms is dissected. No attempt is made to dissect or expose the visceral artery branches. The proximal aortic clamp is slowly applied while cardiac hemodynamics are carefully monitored. Heparin is not used. The distal aortic clamp is then applied. The aneurysm is opened longitudinally in a plane that extends posterior to the origin of the left renal artery. Electrocautery is used to control bleeding from the thickened wall of the aneurysm. IMA, Inferior mesenteric artery; SMA, superior mesenteric artery.

Bleeding from the visceral artery branches is controlled by inserting intraluminal balloon catheters. Although not shown here, perfusion catheters from the atrial-femoral bypass circuit can be inserted both to control back bleeding and provide arterial flow to the viscera. Heavy stay sutures are placed through the aneurysm wall and used for retraction, facilitating exposure of the visceral orifices. Bleeding from intercostal branches is controlled by "figure-of-eight" suture ligation except for large intercostals and lumbars, which are to be reattached to the graft.

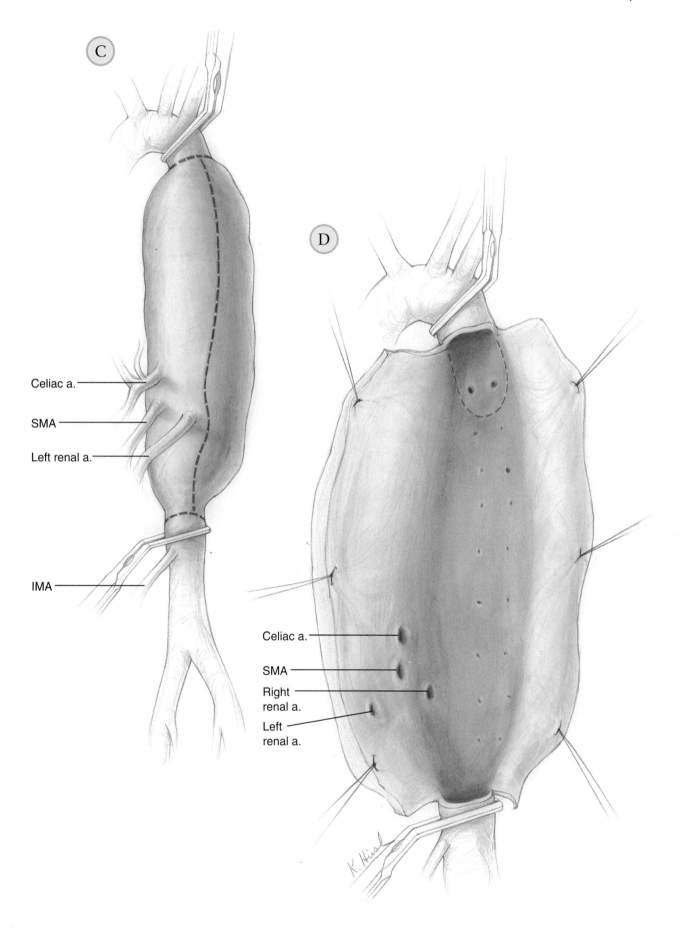

Celiac a.

SMA

Left renal a.

IMA

Celiac a.

SMA

Right renal a.

Left renal a.

A woven Dacron "tube" graft of an appropriate size is selected and anastomosed end-to-end to the proximal uninvolved thoracic aorta using continuous 3–0 monofilament nonabsorbable suture. The back wall is sutured from within the aneurysm. If possible, proximal intercostal orifices are preserved as shown. After completion of the anastomosis, the graft is clamped and the proximal aortic clamp is temporarily released to check the proximal anastomosis. Any suture line bleeding is controlled with interrupted sutures and pledgets as needed.

The graft is stretched under appropriate tension, and an oval opening is made in the side of the graft opposite to visceral ostia. If the ostia are close together, all four can be attached to the graft through one opening. If they are wide apart, separate anastomoses may be necessary. A circumferential anastomosis is performed around the orifices, using a continuous suture placed from within the aneurysm. Large, deep bites should be taken to ensure that full thickness of the aortic wall is incorporated. Occasionally, it may be difficult to attach the left renal artery because of wide separation of the orifices or severe atherosclerotic disease. Reattachment in such cases is performed with a separate 8-mm Dacron graft to the renal artery.

After visceral artery reattachment, air and debris are flushed from the graft by lowering the head of the table and temporarily releasing the proximal aortic clamp. Balloon catheters are removed from the visceral branches, and the graft is clamped distal to the visceral vessels. Care must be exercised to ensure that all air has been evacuated from the large-caliber graft. Flow is then restored to the visceral arteries by slowly removing the proximal aortic clamp while the anesthesiologist rapidly administers blood and crystalloid solution to maintain intravascular volume. The distal anastomosis is then performed in an end-to-end fashion to the normal distal aorta using continuous 3–0 monofilament suture. After completion of this anastomosis, the clamps are removed and the distal aorta is perfused.

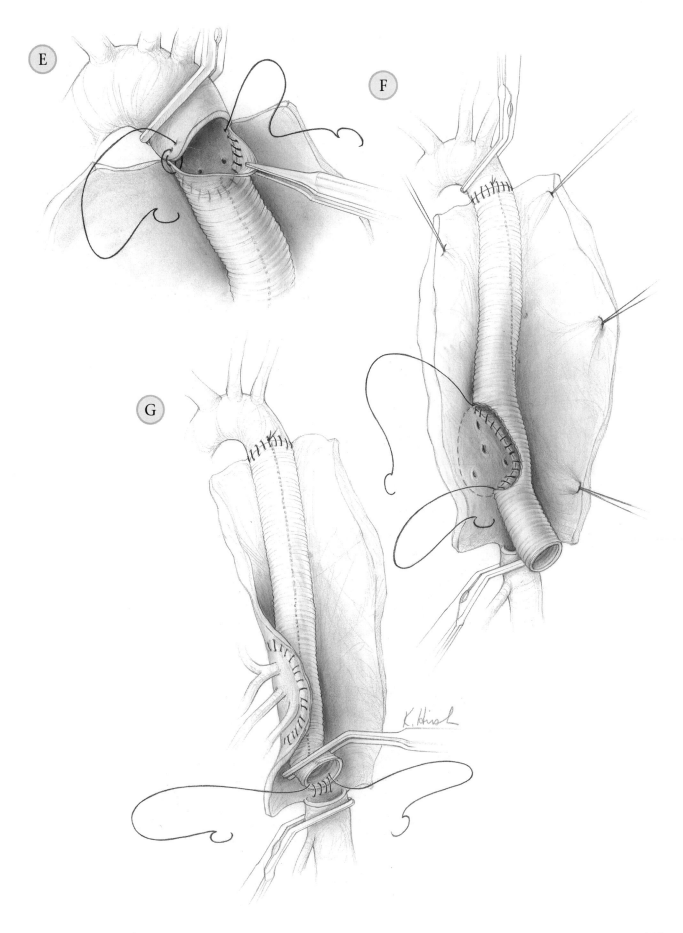

Large intercostal or lumbar arteries, or both, may be anastomosed to the side of the graft to maintain spinal cord blood flow. A vascular clamp is placed on the side of the graft, and an oval opening is made in the graft. A continuous suture line is begun posteriorly and carried around anteriorly, incorporating selected large intercostal arteries. Alternatively, intercostal orifices may be anastomosed to the graft before visceral artery reimplantation (Fig. F, page 129). Unfortunately, there is little evidence that this significantly impacts on the incidence of paraplegia with thoracoabdominal aneurysm repair.

The aneurysm wall is tightly sutured around the aortic reconstruction using a continuous suture to ensure hemostasis and to separate the graft from the lung and adjacent structures. The operation is completed by repair of the diaphragm and closure of the thoracic and abdominal incision. Intercostal chest tube drainage can be limited to a single dependent chest tube if no air leak is demonstrated.

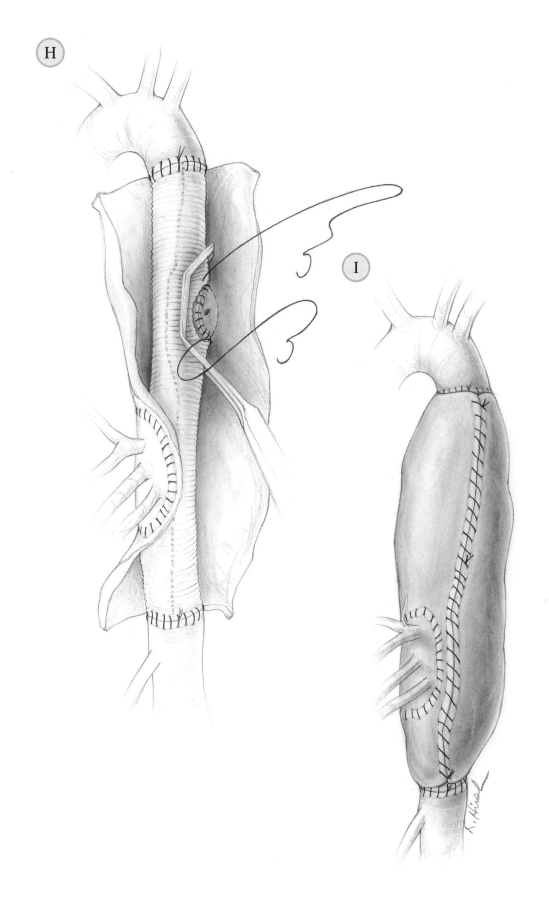

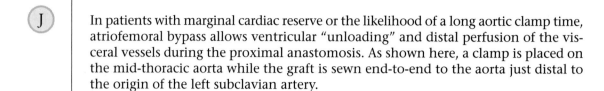

J In patients with marginal cardiac reserve or the likelihood of a long aortic clamp time, atriofemoral bypass allows ventricular "unloading" and distal perfusion of the visceral vessels during the proximal anastomosis. As shown here, a clamp is placed on the mid-thoracic aorta while the graft is sewn end-to-end to the aorta just distal to the origin of the left subclavian artery.

K Following the proximal anastomosis, an "octopus" side arm allows perfusion of the visceral vessels while the Carrel patch is anastomosed as in Figure F.

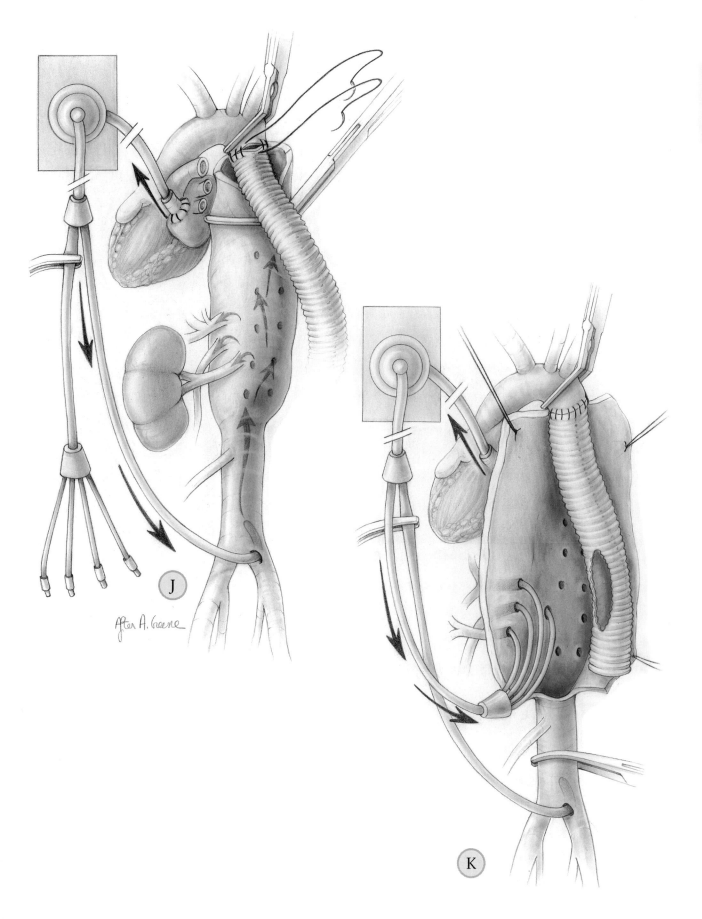

After A. Greene

Femoral Aneurysms

Aneurysms that occur in the groin area may be true aneurysms or false aneurysms, better known as pseudoaneurysms. True atherosclerotic aneurysms in the femoral artery are rare, with an annual incidence of 0.3 per 100,000 patients. Femoral aneurysms usually involve the common femoral artery and are found in elderly male smokers. Most are atherosclerotic in nature and are asymptomatic at the time of diagnosis. Diagnosis is usually made by palpation of the femoral pulse, which becomes prominent and may be visible as a pulsating bulge in thin patients. Diagnosis is confirmed with Duplex ultrasonography, which can define aneurysm size and the presence of mural thombus. Aneurysms larger than 2 cm are considered to be significant, particularly if associated with mural thrombus. Complications include distal embolization (20%), acute thrombosis (15%), and rupture (<10%). Sometimes symptoms are caused by compression of femoral vein or nerve.

Because of the possibility of complications, treatment of large or symptomatic aneurysms is usually indicated. Preoperative evaluation includes visualization of lower extremity arteries with angiography. Alternatively, CT or MR angiography can be used. Surgical repair involves replacement of the aneurysmal femoral artery with a prosthetic graft.

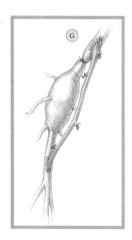

A femoral pseudoaneurysm is a defect in the artery wall caused by an iatrogenic arterial puncture that fails to seal. Femoral artery pseudoaneurysms are more common than true aneurysms because of the high rate of femoral artery punctures for diagnostic arteriograms, arterial pressure monitoring, and endovascular interventional procedures performed through femoral artery access. Femoral artery pseudoaneurysms develop in about 1% of patients undergoing procedures that require femoral cannulation, particularly in patients who are subsequently treated with anticoagulants of antiplatelet agents. Pseudoaneurysms that develop after arterial puncture can be treated with compression under ultrasound guidance, thrombin injection, or open surgical repair. If a patient is hemodynamically unstable, immediate open repair is indicated. Open repair usually requires one or two simple sutures to close the defect in the artery wall.

Pseudoaneurysms may also develop at anastomotic suture lines in the groin, such as after aortofemoral bypass or femoropopliteal bypass. Anastomotic pseudoaneurysms may develop as a result of mechanical failure of the suture or graft fabric in areas of stress, trauma, or tension. Such pseudoaneurysms may be repaired by replacing the graft or repairing the defect. Some pseudoaneurysms develop as a result of infection in the graft material and/or infection and dissolution of the artery wall. Under these circumstances, the vascular graft must be removed, the infected artery wall debrided and ligated, and the extraanatomic bypass established to restore blood flow around the infected area.

A vertical incision is made in the groin directly over the aneurysm. Control of the proximal common femoral artery is obtained just below the inguinal ligament. If necessary, the inguinal ligament may be divided to obtain better exposure. For very large aneurysms, proximal control may be obtained above the inguinal ligament through a transverse suprainguinal incision. The proximal superficial femoral and profunda femoris arteries are controlled distal to the aneurysm.

Vascular clamps are applied to the proximal external iliac artery and distal superficial femoral and profunda arteries, and the aneurysm is opened using a longitudinal arteriotomy. Mural thrombus is removed. The neck of the aneurysm may be totally transected or left intact posteriorly. An 8- or 10-mm prosthetic graft is selected and anastomosed end-to-end to the proximal common femoral artery using 4–0 or 5–0 monofilament vascular suture. Dacron or polytetrafluoroethylene grafts are equally suitable. The graft is trimmed to a suitable length and anastomosed to the femoral bifurcation with 5–0 suture taking care to preserve flow to both the superficial femoral and profunda arteries. Orifice endarterectomies may be performed, or the graft may be extended onto the distal vessels as necessary.

If the superficial femoral artery is totally occluded and there is extensive atherosclerosis at the origin of the profunda, the arteriotomy should be extended until normal profunda lumen is reached. If needed, endarterectomy is performed and the graft is anastomosed end-to-end to the profunda.

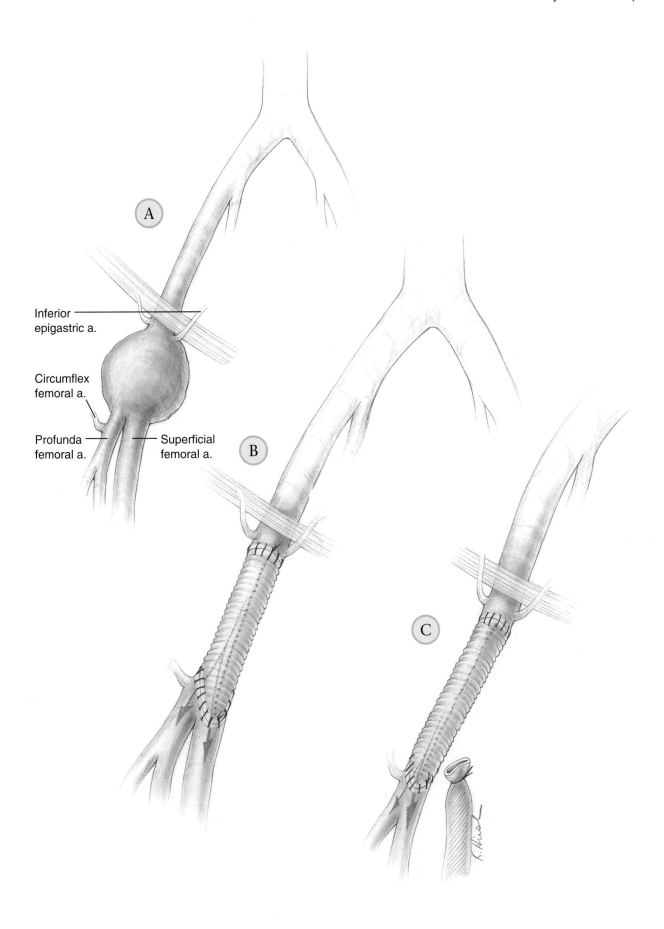

Inferior
epigastric a.

Circumflex
femoral a.

Profunda
femoral a.

Superficial
femoral a.

A

B

C

Popliteal Aneurysms

Popliteal aneurysms are the most common peripheral arterial aneurysm. The prevalence rate of popliteal aneurysms in men older than 65 years is approximately 1%, whereas the prevalence is much greater in men with abdominal aortic aneurysm (14%). Men who have a popliteal aneurysm have a high likelihood (50%) of having an abdominal aortic aneurysm, and popliteal aneurysms are bilateral in 70% of patients. Thus, all men with a popliteal aneurysm should undergo abdominal ultrasound to screen for abdominal aortic aneurysm and ultrasound examination of the opposite popliteal artery. The close relation between popliteal aneurysm and abdominal aortic aneurysm is not seen in women. In women, with or without abdominal aortic aneurysm, popliteal aneurysm is rare.

Rupture of popliteal aneurysms is uncommon. The most common clinical complication of popliteal aneurysm is thrombosis, distal thromboembolism, or both, often leading to limb-threatening ischemia. Other clinical signs include pain or weakness from tibial nerve compression and swelling or deep vein thrombosis from popliteal vein compression. Only one third of patients with popliteal aneurysm who are treated conservatively remain free of symptoms or complications at 5 years. Popliteal aneurysm is often diagnosed by palpation of the pulsating or thrombosed mass in the popliteal fossa. Sometimes popliteal aneurysm may be confused with a Baker's cyst in the popliteal fossa. Duplex ultrasonography is the best initial study for the evaluation of popliteal aneurysm size and to determine if mural thrombus is present. Popliteal aneurysms greater than 2 cm in diameter are considered to be significant, particularly if associated with mural thrombus. Duplex ultrasound is also the examination of choice for acute popliteal occlusion when previously undiagnosed popliteal aneurysmal disease is suspected. Angiography is essential in evaluating popliteal aneurysms to demonstrate the extent of the involved segment and to evaluate the patency and quality of the runoff vessels and to detect distal embolic occlusions. Aneurysm size, however, cannot be reliably measured from angiography because of intramural thrombus. Angiography also offers the opportunity to perform thrombolysis in patients with acute popliteal thrombosis.

Popliteal aneurysms are best treated by opening the aneurysm, evacuating the mural thrombus, suture-ligating geniculate branches from within the aneurysm, and placing an interposition reversed vein bypass within the aneurysm sac to restore flow. Alternatively, the aneurysm may be ligated and bypassed from a normal segment of the superficial femoral artery to the distal popliteal or tibial artery. In case of distal thromboembolism, thromboembolectomy or thrombolysis may be necessary to establish distal arterial runoff.

Death after repair of femoral and popliteal aneurysms is rare, and limb salvage rates in asymptomatic patients are 90% to 98%. In symptomatic patients, early graft patency rate is 59% to 85%, and the limb salvage rate is 70% to 80%. Patients who experience thrombosis of untreated popliteal aneurysms have a limb loss rate of 50%.

Popliteal artery aneurysms may cause ischemia of the lower extremity by thrombosis of the aneurysms or embolization of mural thrombus to the distal circulation. Although popliteal aneurysms rupture only rarely, symptoms may arise by compression of the adjacent popliteal vein or tibial nerve. The diagnosis can usually be made by palpation of the pulsating or thrombosed mass in the popliteal fossa. Duplex ultrasound imaging confirms the diagnosis. Femoral arteriography is essential before popliteal aneurysm repair to delineate the patency of the popliteal trifurcation and outflow vessels.

D   If the popliteal aneurysm is totally thrombosed with a patent superficial femoral artery proximally and a patent popliteal trifurcation or tibial artery distally, bypass of the aneurysm using a saphenous vein is the procedure of choice. The selection of proximal and distal anastomotic sites are based on the femoral arteriogram. Incisions are made over the patent distal superficial femoral artery and over the popliteal trifurcation (see page 249). An appropriate length of saphenous vein is harvested from the medial thigh.

E   A tunnel is created through the popliteal fossa using blunt dissection.

F   The saphenous vein bypass may be reversed or transposed. We prefer to use the vein transposed so that the large proximal portion of the vein is anastomosed to the large superficial femoral artery and the smaller distal vein is matched in size to the smaller popliteal or tibial artery. The proximal vein is cannulated and flushed retrograde with heparinized saline to close the valves. A valvulotome is introduced through the end of the vein and each valve lysed (see page 243).

G   The vein bypass is anastomosed end-to-end or end-to-side proximally and distally using 5–0 monofilament nonabsorbable suture. The superficial femoral artery distal to the proximal anastomosis is ligated to prevent distal embolization from the aneurysm or proximal propagation of thrombus into the anastomosis or both. The popliteal artery distal to the aneurysm may be left unligated if large geniculate arteries are present to maintain flow. That said, if the popliteal aneurysm is large, it may cause compression of the popliteal vein and tibial nerve. It is then preferable to ligate all obvious branches, open the aneurysm to evacuate the mural thrombus, and suture ligate any back bleeding vessels from within the decompressed aneurysm sac.

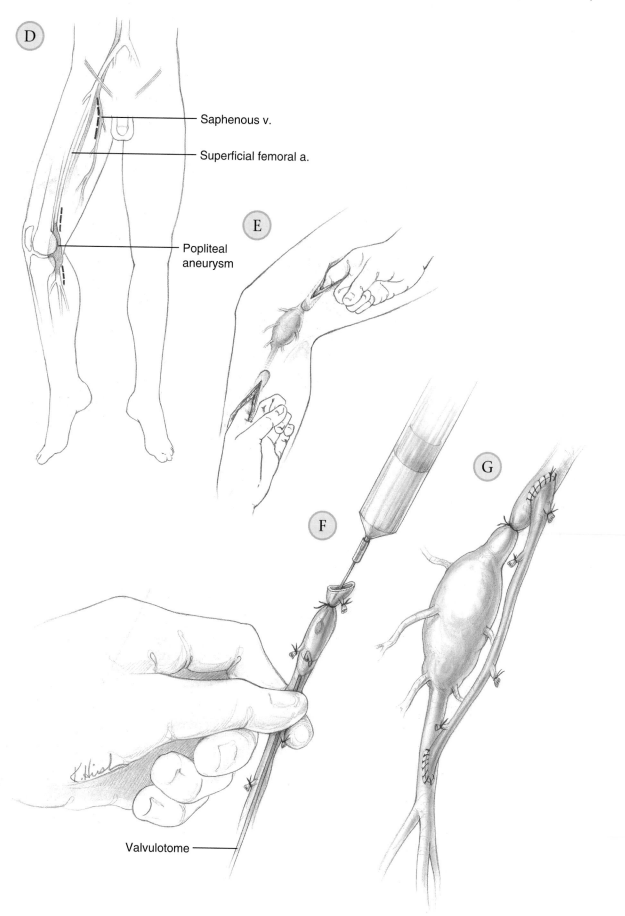

D

Saphenous v.

Superficial femoral a.

E

Popliteal
aneurysm

F

G

Valvulotome

Extensive Femoral Aneurysmosis

Patients with aneurysmosis have enlargement of most or all major arteries including the aorta and lower extremity arteries. The majority of patients are asymptomatic, and the true incidence is unknown. Patients may have involvement of the infrarenal aorta, iliac, and common femoral arteries (type I), isolated femoral and popliteal aneurysms with arteriomegaly of the superficial femoral artery (type II), or the more frequently occurring combination of the previous two types (type III). Possible explanations for this pathology are a generalized disorder of connective tissue. However, patients usually have no identifiable connective tissue disorder. Clinical presentation is commonly that of an isolated peripheral aneurysm with the discovery of multiple ectatic and aneurysmal arteries with further examination. Arteriography, ultrasonography, and abdominal CT scan are instrumental in diagnosing the scope of disease. Patients with diffuse ectasia and aneurysmosis appear to be somewhat less likely to sustain rupture than patients with isolated focal aneurysmal disease of the same diameter. The treatment of patients with aneurysmosis should be dictated by the presenting symptoms and aneurysm size. Surgical interventions and treatments should be selected so that the most life-threatening disease is addressed first. In most of these patients, femoral and popliteal aneurysms are present.

(H) When the entire superficial femoropopliteal vessel is aneurysmal, a bypass must be constructed from the nonaneurysmal proximal femoral artery to a patent distal tibial artery. This is best accomplished with a saphenous vein bypass. Incisions are made in the medial thigh and popliteal fossa to expose the normal superficial femoral or common femoral artery and the popliteal artery (see pages 227–229). The saphenous vein is harvested from the contralateral leg, and valve cusps are lysed (see page 243) to render them incompetent. The translocated saphenous vein is tunnelled deep to the sartorius muscle from the femoral artery to the popliteal fossa.

(I) The large proximal saphenous vein is anastomosed end-to-side to the normal femoral artery, and the distal vein is anastomosed to the tibial artery. The aneurysmal segment is excluded by ligatures proximally and distally. A completion arteriogram is obtained to demonstrate the bypass graft, anastomosis, and outflow vessels. If the aneurysm has caused venous or neural compression, it is necessary to decompress the aneurysm after the bypass. The medial aspect of the aneurysm is exposed in the popliteal fossa with great care to avoid injury to surrounding veins and nerves. The aneurysmal sac is incised and the orifices of geniculate arteries and the distal superficial femoral artery are oversewn from within. The aneurysmal sac is left open.

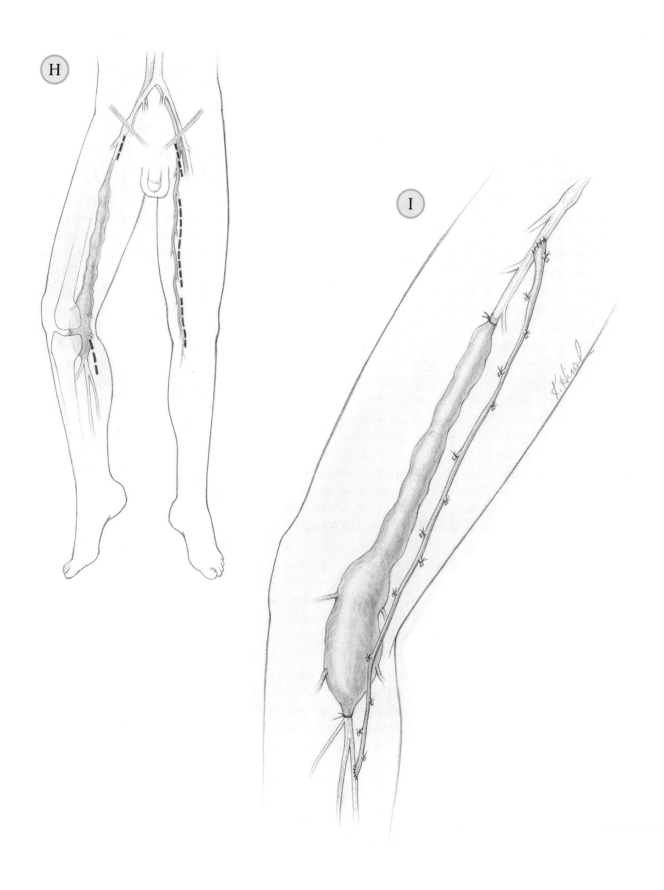

SECTION III

Renal Revascularization

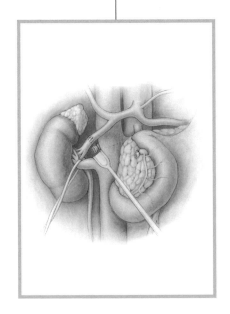

Although renovascular disease is a relatively rare cause of hypertension (1–5% of adults with hypertension), it is the most common surgically correctable cause. Renovascular disease in the elderly is caused primarily by atherosclerotic narrowing of the renal arteries and may result in both progressive hypertension and diminished renal function. In younger patients, especially children and women between 20 and 35 years of age, renovascular disease is most commonly caused by fibromuscular dysplasia. Clinical features that increase the likelihood of a renovascular cause of hypertension include new onset of hypertension, rapid progression of previously stable hypertension, and hypertension associated with renal function impairment.

A more aggressive approach in the treatment of renovascular disease has resulted from three recent developments: (1) an increased recognition of ischemic nephropathy as an important consequence of renovascular disease separate from hypertension; (2) the widespread acceptance of percutaneous renal angioplasty; and (3) improved results of surgical revascularization. Currently accepted indications for renal revascularization include the presence of a hemodynamically significant renal artery stenosis (> 60% diameter) in patients with refractory hypertension or hypertension associated with renal functional impairment. In recent reports, substantial improvements in renal function have been noted even in patients older than 65 years with significant and progressive azotemia (serum creatinine > 4 mg/dl). Renal Duplex scanning has evolved into the principal noninvasive screening test for both the presence of renal arterial disease and its hemodynamic significance. The modality combines B-mode ultrasound imaging with pulsed Doppler ultrasound determinations of blood flow velocity. The ratio of renal artery peak systolic velocity to aortic peak systolic velocity (RAR) has been used to define hemodynamically significant lesions. Lesions of 60% or greater are associated with RAR of greater than 3.5.

Arteriography is still the accepted standard for diagnosis of renovascular disease. Multiple views of the renal vessels are obtained including, at least, anteroposterior and oblique views. The measurement of renal vein renin levels has been used as an adjunct to arteriography to help identify functionally significant renal arterial stenoses. Such values can be expressed as renal vein renin ratios, which compare one kidney with the other (ratios > 1.5 are considered diagnostic), or renal/systemic renin indices, which quantify the contribution of each kidney to the total systemic renin level.

Percutaneous renal angioplasty has been a prominent form of modern therapy in both atherosclerotic and fibromuscular lesions of the renal artery. Previously, the success of these interventions was limited by a relatively high recurrence rate and inability to apply angioplasty in orificial atherosclerotic lesions, which are the most common lesions encountered. The more recent development of self-expanding and balloon-expandable stents has demonstrated better outcomes for these lesions. That said, operative repair remains an important option in these patients, especially those who have lesions that are not amenable to angioplasty because they involve the distal portion of the renal artery or those with recurrent disease after angioplasty. Furthermore, open surgical intervention may be a better option in patients with ischemic nephropathy in which salvage of renal parenchyma is the primary indication.

Surgical options include endarterectomy and aortorenal or hepatorenal bypasses. Endarterectomy through a transaortic route is most useful in bilateral orificial disease, but it requires suprarenal aortic exposure and clamping with resultant greater cardiac risk. Aortorenal bypass from a relatively disease-free area of the infrarenal aorta has been the most widely used technique in the past, although hepatorenal and splenorenal bypasses are currently used more frequently. The latter procedures avoid manipulation of the often diseased aorta and obviates any need for aortic occlusion.

Irrespective of the origin of these bypass grafts, long-term patency is excellent, approaching 95% over 5 years if autogenous vein is used. In a recent series of 35 patients older than 60 years, improvement or cure of hypertension was reported in 90% of patients and improvement in renal function in more than a third. Overall morbidity and mortality rates in this group (5% mortality, 20% perioperative morbidity) appeared to be related to generalized atherosclerosis and accompanying risk factors.

A number of surgical approaches have been described to revascularize renal arteries obstructed by atherosclerosis or fibromuscular dysplasia. These include aortorenal bypass, endarterectomy, renal artery reimplantation, segmental renal artery resection with reanastomosis, splenorenal or hepatorenal anastomosis, and renal autotransplantation. Although no single technique is applicable to all situations and any one of these techniques may be superior in any given patient, the procedure we have found to be most widely applicable is the aortorenal bypass with autogenous saphenous vein. Other conduits are also acceptable; autogenous hypogastric artery may be considered in children, and prosthetic bypasses may be used in renal artery bypasses performed in conjunction with prosthetic aortic grafts.

Adequate exposure of the renal arteries is the most important aspect of renal artery surgery. Exposure of both renal arteries can be obtained transperitoneally through a midline incision. However, better visualization and control can be obtained through a flank or transverse incision. For the left renal artery, we prefer a retroperitoneal approach. A transperitoneal approach using a supraumbilical transverse incision is preferred for the right renal artery.

A bean bag is used to position the patient on the operating table with the left shoulder at a 45-degree angle and the left arm suspended in a sling. A supraumbilical transverse incision is made and extended to the tip of the twelfth rib. The internal and external oblique muscles and left rectus muscle are divided. The fibers of the transversus abdominus are split, and the peritoneum is mobilized from the costal margin to the iliac crest.

The peritoneum is retracted to the right, and the ureter and iliopsoas muscles are identified. The retroperitoneal plane between the left colon and kidney is developed to expose the testicular vein and left renal vein. The left renal vein is mobilized, and control is obtained of the infrarenal abdominal aorta between the level of the renal arteries and inferior mesenteric artery (IMA). The kidney is not mobilized or removed from Gerota's capsule so that collateral blood supply is preserved.

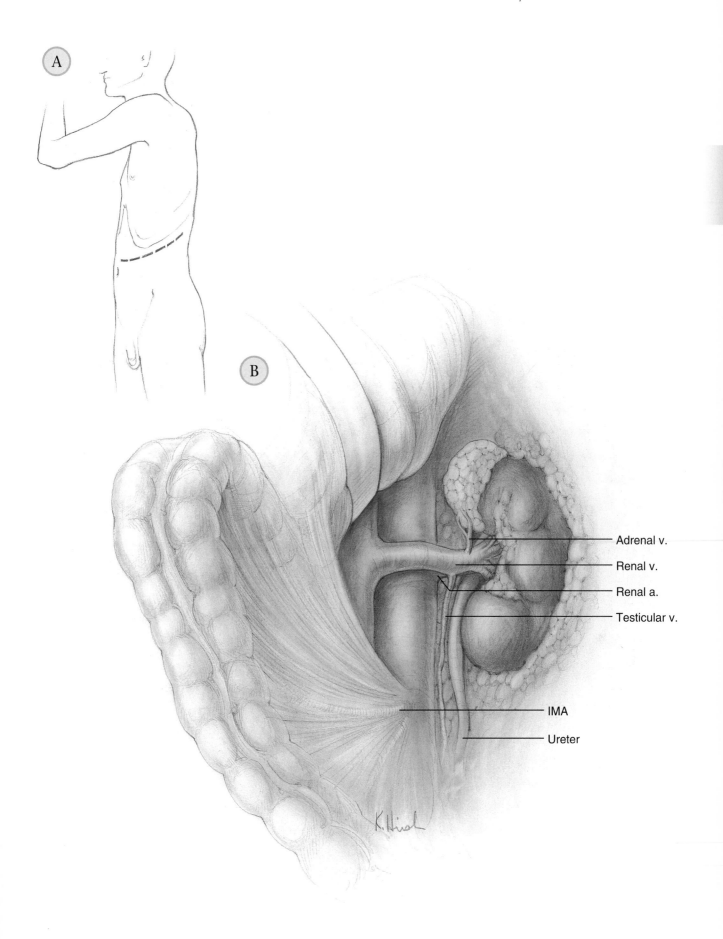

Adrenal v.

Renal v.

Renal a.

Testicular v.

IMA

Ureter

C

The left renal vein is retracted superiorly exposing the underlying left renal artery. The testicular vein is divided and ligated to facilitate exposure. Control is obtained of the renal artery distal to the obstructing lesion. To minimize renal ischemia time, the saphenous vein bypass is first anastomosed to the infrarenal aorta. After systemic heparinization, the aorta is clamped. If the aorta is soft and does not have significant atherosclerosis, a partial occlusion clamp is used so that flow is maintained to the lower extremities. If the aorta is severely diseased, cross-clamping the aorta with two vascular clamps will provide better exposure of the aorta for anastomosis and the opportunity to perform local aortic endarterectomy. The aorta is opened with a longitudinal aortotomy, and the luminal surface is inspected.

D

The saphenous vein, previously harvested from the thigh, is reversed and anastomosed to the infrarenal aorta using 5–0 or 6–0 continuous monofilament suture. The vein is spatulated to prevent anastomotic stenosis.

E

The aortic clamp is released to flush out any atherosclerotic debris before completion of the suture line.

F

Direct anastomosis of a small saphenous vein to an extensively diseased and calcified aorta should be avoided. A larger than normal aortotomy should be made and a saphenous vein patch sewn in place using 4–0 or 5–0 continuous suture. Large bites can be made in the aorta to avoid calcified areas. An opening is then made in the center of the vein patch and the reversed saphenous vein anastomosed to the vein patch using 6–0 continuous suture. The aorta is unclamped, the graft is flushed, and a Heifetz vascular clamp is applied to the vein graft for hemostasis during the distal anastomosis.

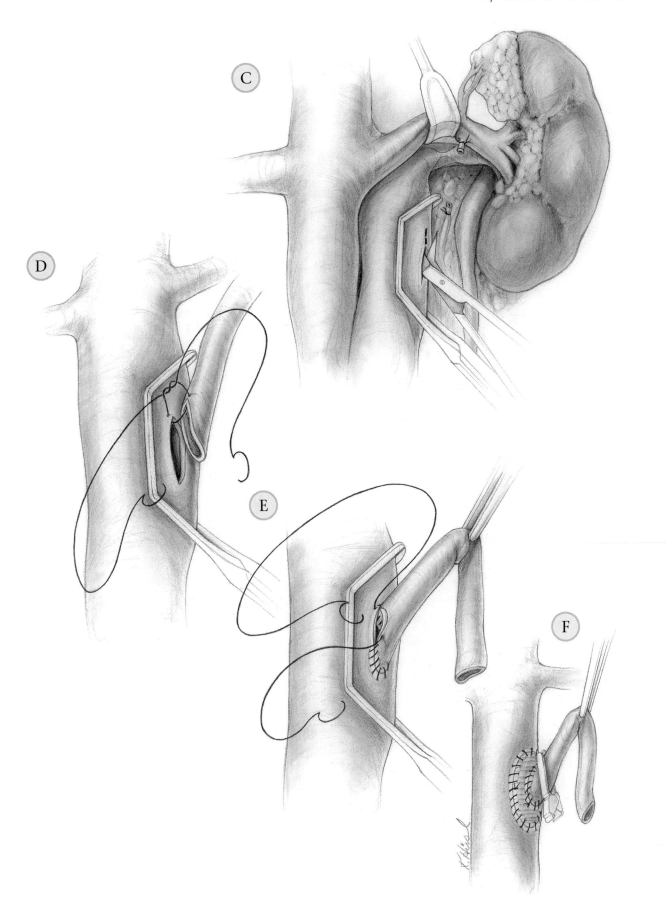

C

D

E

F

An atraumatic vascular clamp is placed on the distal renal artery, and the proximal renal artery is clamped and transected distal to the obstructing lesion. The distal renal artery is flushed with cold, heparinized balanced salt solution. The proximal renal artery stump is suture ligated. If sufficient renal artery is available, a segment of renal artery may be sent to pathology for examination. The distal renal artery is cut longitudinally on its anterior surface for at least the length of the vessel diameter. The clamp on the saphenous vein is released and the distal vein graft is pinched to ascertain proper length and orientation of the vein relative to the renal artery.

The saphenous vein is cut to appropriate length and spatulated to match the renal artery. The anastomosis is begun by placing 6–0 monofilament suture at the 6 and 12 o'clock positions using loupe magnification to ensure precision. Both sutures are tied, and care is taken to avoid undue tension that may tear the renal artery. One side of the anastomosis is then completed with continuous suture running from the vein to the artery.

The anastomosis is rotated and the other side is completed. Before completion of the anastomosis, the proximal and distal clamps are temporarily released to flush out air and debris. Satisfactory flow through the vein graft is confirmed by palpation of the pulse and Doppler ultrasound signals in the graft and distal renal artery.

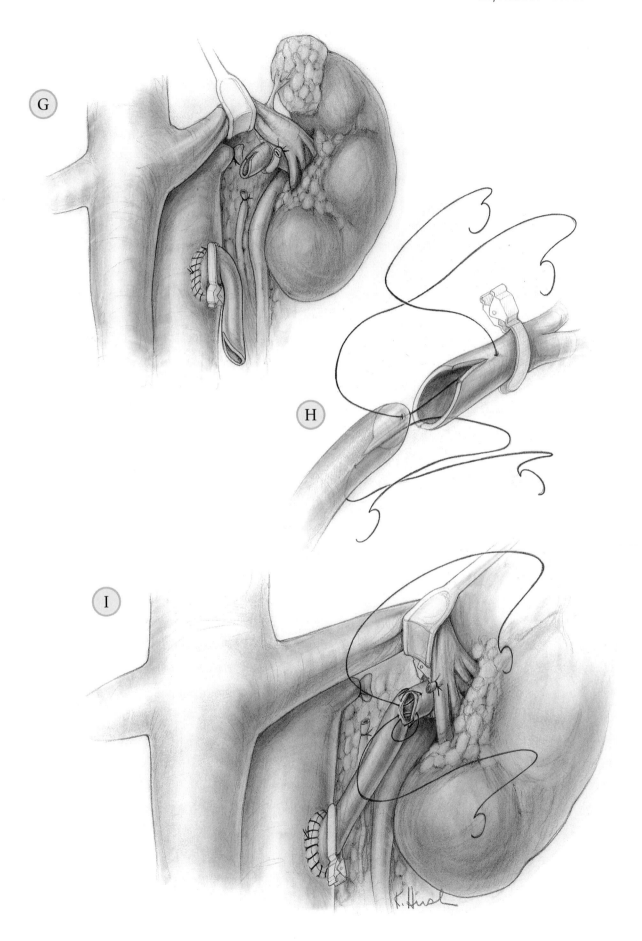

Exposure of the right renal artery is obtained through a transverse supraumbilical incision extending from the midline to the right flank. The duodenum and right colon are mobilized to the midline exposing the right renal vein and vena cava. Care should be taken to avoid avulsion of the gonadal vein, which enters the anterior surface of the inferior vena cava. The right renal vein and right side of the inferior vena cava are mobilized. The right renal artery lies behind and superior to the renal vein and is mobilized and encircled with silastic tapes. The inferior vena cava is dissected free of the infrarenal aorta, and a segment of soft infrarenal aorta is exposed. The vena cava is mobilized posteriorly between the aorta and renal artery along the course of the aortorenal bypass. Lumbar veins are carefully identified, ligated, and divided, if necessary, for mobilization of the vena cava. The saphenous vein is harvested from the thigh.

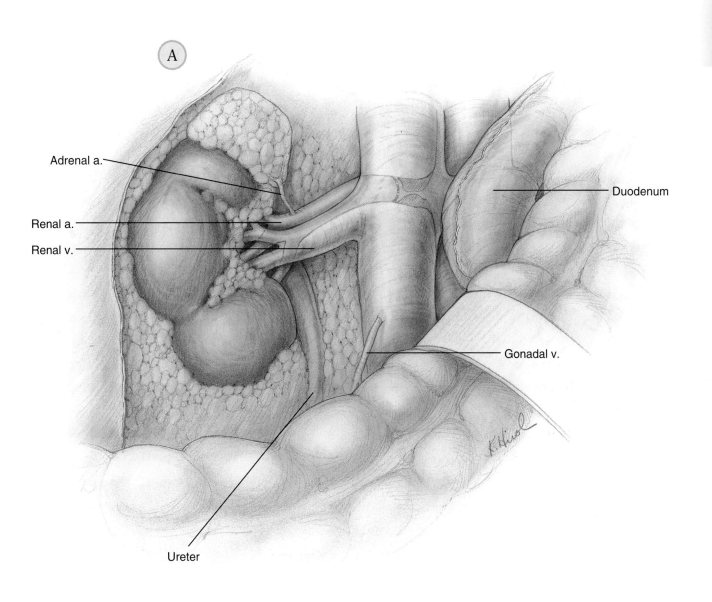

A

Adrenal a.

Renal a.

Renal v.

Duodenum

Gonadal v.

Ureter

After systemic heparinization, the proximal renal artery is clamped and transected. The distal renal artery is flushed with cold, heparinized balanced salt solution, and the distal renal artery is occluded with a Heifetz clip. If the main renal artery is extensively diseased, it may be necessary to individually control and clamp the branches of the renal artery. The proximal renal artery is suture ligated. The distal renal artery is opened longitudinally on its anterior surface and is spatulated to enlarge the anastomotic area and to ensure that there is no residual occlusive disease at or distal to the anastomotic location. The reversed saphenous vein is anastomosed end-to-end to the distal renal artery using two 6–0 monofilament vascular sutures placed under loupe magnification. The saphenous vein is carefully tunneled underneath the vena cava for anastomosis to the aorta. The aorta is usually soft and may be clamped using a partial occluding clamp. If the aorta has significant atherosclerosis, total occlusion of the aortic segment using two vascular clamps provides better exposure for the anastomosis. The aortotomy is performed on the anterolateral right side of the aorta to achieve the best lie of the graft.

The saphenous vein is cut to appropriate length and tailored to match the size of the aortotomy. The anasotomisis is performed using a single continuous monofilament suture. The suture is begun in the center of the back wall and run in both directions. Before completion of the suture line on the anterior wall, the aorta is flushed and the distal renal artery clamp is removed to permit back bleeding. Flow in the graft and distal renal artery is checked by palpation of the pulse and Doppler ultrasound.

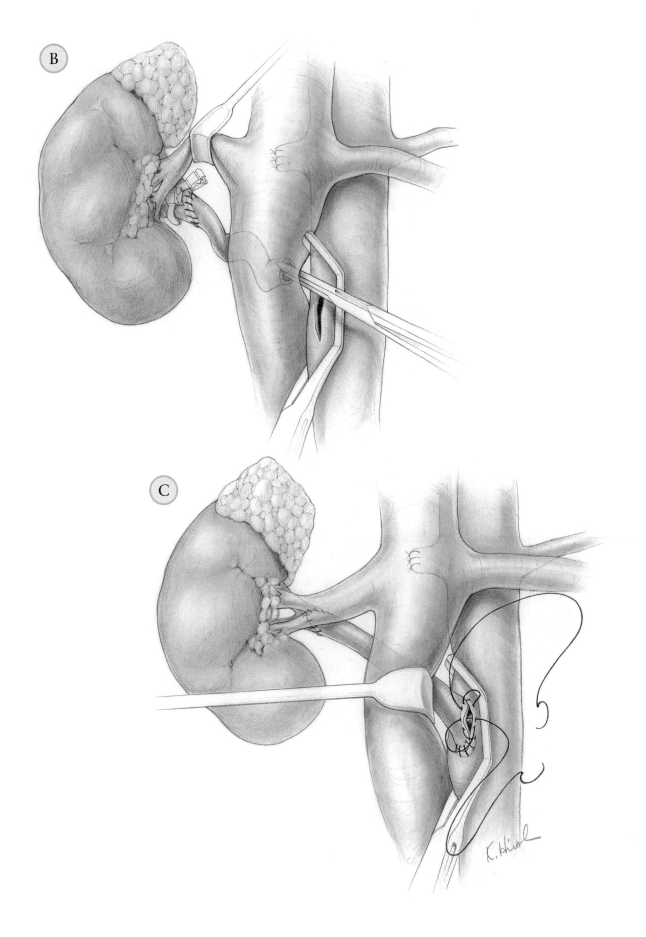

In patients with previous aortic surgery or with advanced aortoiliac disease, hepatorenal bypass offers the possibility of successful revascularization of the kidney without the difficulties of repeat aortic exposure or the stress of aortic occlusion. Attention must be directed to the lateral views of the celiac axis and its branches on aortogram to ensure that there is no inflow lesion of the celiac artery.

 After a generous Kocher maneuver, the hepatic artery is exposed. The preferred site of a proximal anastomosis is distal to the origin of the gastroduodenal artery. A vein graft of the hypogastric artery is the ideal conduit. Proximal anastomosis is performed in an end-to-side fashion to the hepatic artery, and a relatively short graft is placed to the more distal aspect of the right renal artery.

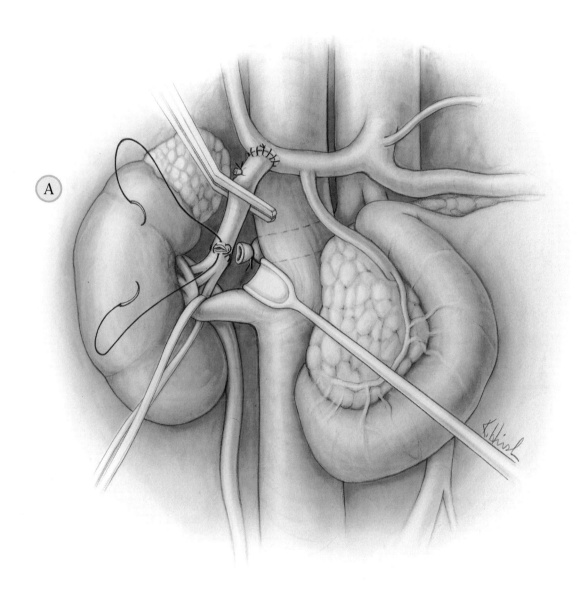

Alternatively, if the gastroduodenal artery is of large caliber (> 3 mm), the artery can be transected at its most distal point and sewn to the right renal artery in an end-to-end fashion.

If there is a size discrepancy between the gastroduodenal and renal artery or if transection of the renal artery would make exposure and stabilization of the distal anastomotic site more difficult, an end-to-side anastomosis can be carried out.

End-to-end

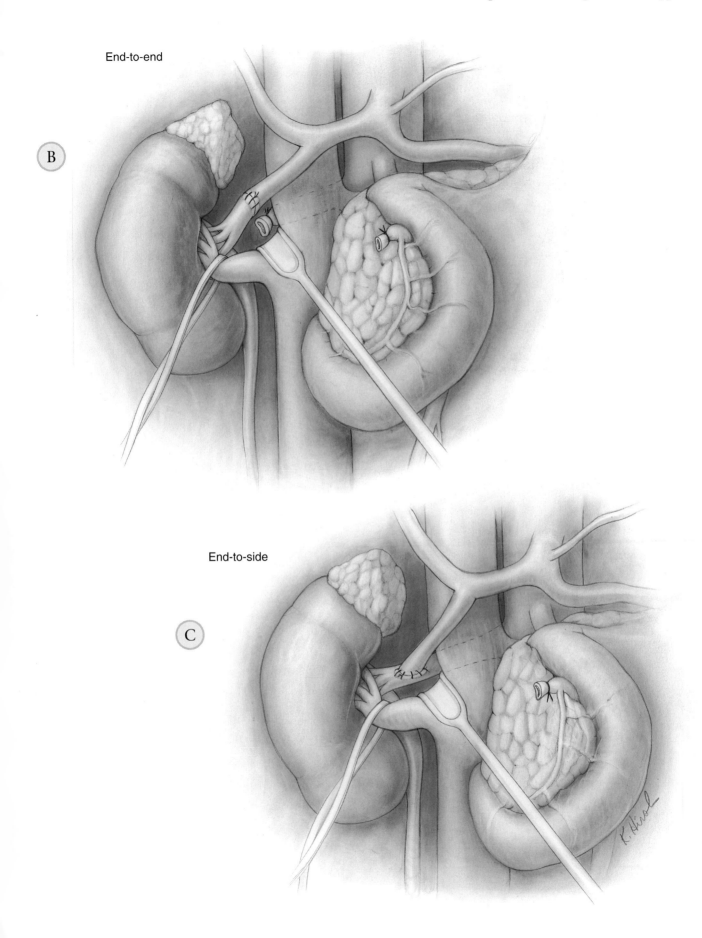

End-to-side

For left renal revascularization, similar surgical techniques can be used with the splenic artery as an inflow vessel. Multiple branches of the splenic artery are ligated, allowing mobilization of the transected splenic artery to the left renal artery. As shown here, an end-to-end anastomosis can be performed. Similarly, an end-to-side anastomosis can also be used. In general, splenorenal bypasses are more difficult than hepatorenal bypass because the splenic artery can be more fragile and has multiple branches requiring some mobilization from the pancreas.

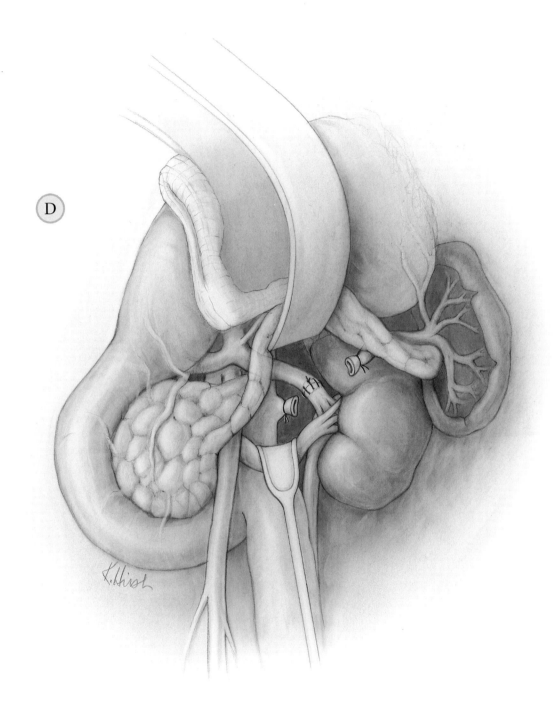

A   Renal artery stenoses involving the branch renal arteries in the hilum of the kidney may be difficult to visualize and to repair *in situ*. In these unusual circumstances, it may be best to temporarily remove the kidney from the abdomen so that the lesions can be better visualized and more precisely corrected.

B   A vascular clamp is placed on the proximal renal vein, and the proximal renal artery is suture ligated. The renal artery and vein are transected, and the kidney is gently lifted from its fossa leaving the ureter intact.

C   The renal artery is flushed with cold, heparinized balanced salt solution until the venous effluent is clear.

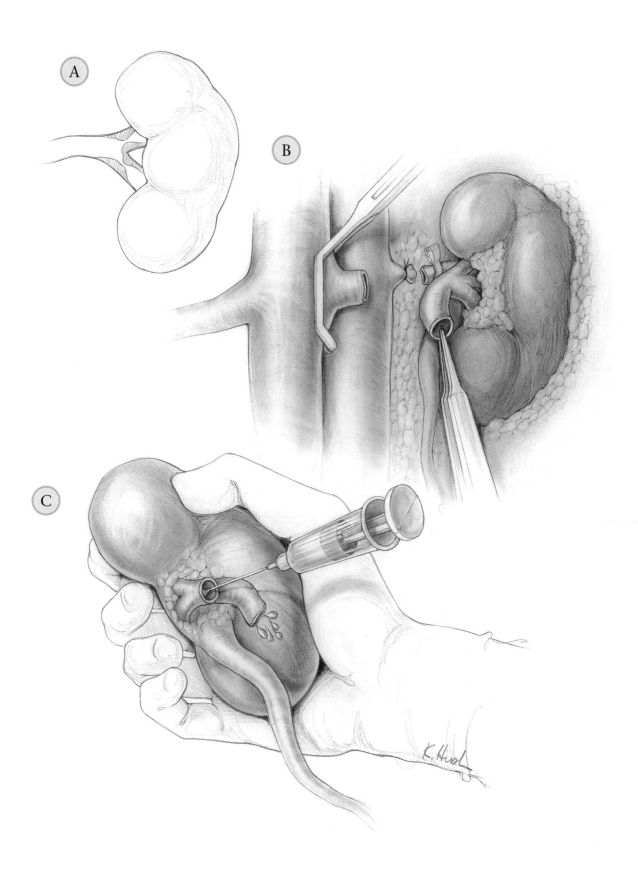

D   The kidney is placed on a plastic sheet in a basin filled with ice. The renal artery branches in the hilum of the kidney are carefully dissected under magnification and lesions are identified. Renal artery branches are opened as necessary to expose all lesions.

E   The reversed saphenous vein is then tailored for the anastomosis to the renal artery branches. The anastomosis is performed using continuous 6–0 or 7–0 monofilament suture under magnification. The kidney is replaced into the renal fossa, and the saphenous vein is anastomosed to the infrarenal aorta. A Heifetz clip is maintained on the saphenous vein, and the kidney is not perfused until completion of the venous anastomosis.

F   The left renal vein is anastomosed using three 6–0 sutures tied at 10, 2, and 6 o'clock (triangulation) to avoid "purse-string" stenosis. After completion of the venous anastomosis, flow is restored to the renal artery. Patency of the bypass is confirmed by immediate return of color to the kidney, fill of the renal vein, and Doppler flow signals in the branch renal arteries.

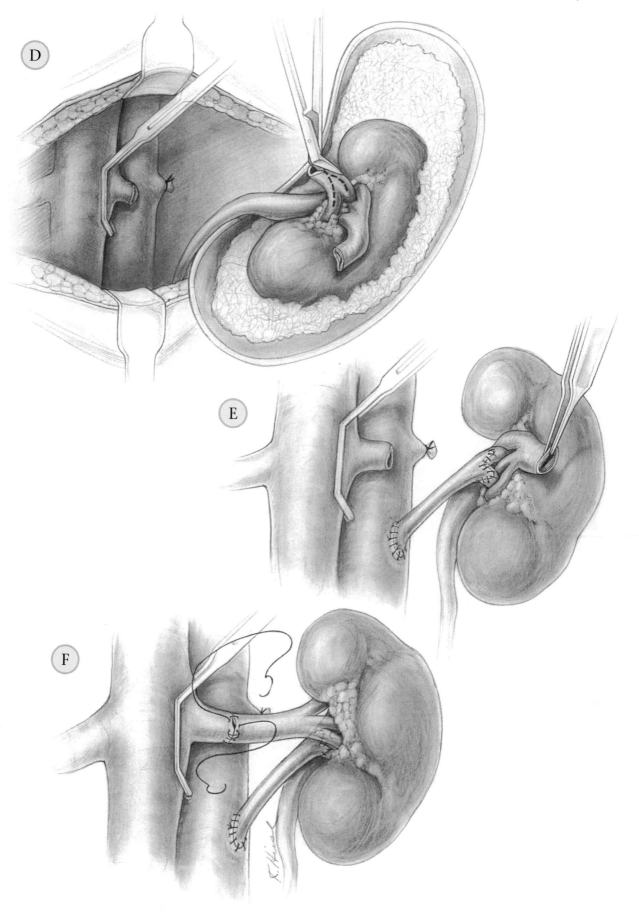

Patients with severe hypertension or deteriorating renal function, or both, who have severe renal artery stenosis may benefit from renal revascularization in association with aortic reconstruction.

(A) If the renal artery stenosis is limited to the orifice and there is a sufficiently long renal artery, it may be possible to reimplant the vessel directly into the aortic graft. After completion of the aortic procedure, the left renal artery is suture ligated and transected. The distal renal artery is flushed with cold, heparinized balanced salt solution and clamped with a Heifetz clip. The renal artery is mobilized, and a suitable location on the aortic graft is identified. The aortic graft is partially occluded with a vascular clamp, and a window is excised from the graft. The renal artery is anastomosed to the aortic graft using a 6–0 continuous suture.

(B) If the renal artery is too short for direct implantation into the aortic graft, an interposition graft is sutured end-to-end to the distal renal artery and anastomosed end-to-side to the body of the aortic graft. Saphenous vein or a short-length (6 mm) prosthetic graft may be used.

(C) As an alternative technique, one renal artery can be excised with a cuff of aorta, as shown here. The proximal anastomosis is then carried obliquely above the level of the left renal artery. The left renal artery and aortic patch are then reimplanted into the side of the aortic graft. The suprarenal clamp is removed as soon as the proximal anastomoses are completed and replaced below the renal arteries.

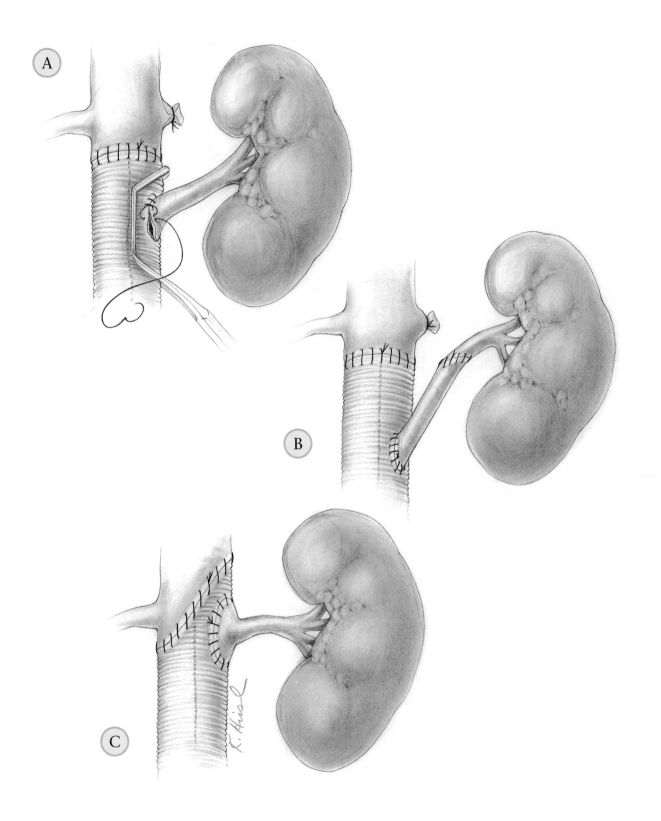

SECTION IV

Mesenteric Revascularization

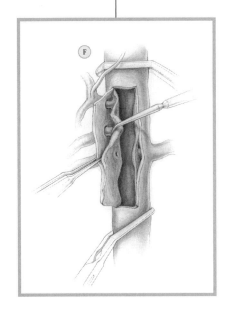

Acute Mesenteric Ischemia

Acute mesenteric ischemia usually occurs in patients older than 70 years who may also have other systemic illnesses, especially gastrointestinal, peripheral vascular, and coronary artery disease. These concomitant factors may color the presentation of the problem and contribute to the frequent delays in diagnosis; such serious comorbidity also decreases the likelihood of successful treatment.

The classic presentation of acute mesenteric ischemia is abdominal pain out of proportion to physical findings. The pain is usually steady, severe, and midabdominal. If peritoneal signs are elicited, it is likely that intestinal infarction has already occurred. The occurrence of bowel infarction greatly increases mortality and morbidity. In some series, infarction is associated with a greater than 80% mortality rate. This fact underscores the importance of early diagnosis and treatment of acute ischemia and expeditious arterial reconstructions in chronic ischemia before acute ischemia supervenes.

One of the most frequently encountered causes of acute ischemia is embolism, which accounts for about one third of all mesenteric vascular catastrophes. Most emboli occur in association with cardiac arrhythmias (especially atrial tachyarrhythmias) or myocardial infarctions. The superior mesenteric artery (SMA) is the site of most embolic occlusions because of its near parallel course to the abdominal aorta.

Acute thrombosis of an already compromised vessel lumen occurs in another one third of cases. Such preexisting atherosclerotic lesions are often associated with prodromal symptoms. In fact, more than 50% of patients with acute SMA thrombosis have a history of postprandial abdominal pain and weight loss. Intestinal angina typically occurs 15 to 60 minutes after meals and is more closely correlated with the volume of food consumed rather than any specific type of food. *In situ* thrombosis typically occurs at the origin of the SMA resulting in gut infarction from the proximal jejunum to the midtransverse colon.

Other causes of mesenteric ischemia are nonocclusive vasospasm and mesenteric venous thrombosis. These entities are usually not treated surgically other than resection of nonviable bowel.

The clinician's single greatest tool for the successful diagnosis of an acute mesenteric vascular event is a high index of suspicion in patients with multiple risk factors. Although many laboratory abnormalities occur with mesenteric ischemia and infarction, most are nonspecific, and thus not diagnostic. These abnormalities include hemoconcentration, leukocytosis with a "left shift," metabolic acidosis, hyperamylasemia, and hyperphosphatemia.

Abdominal roentgenograms are useful in excluding other causes of abdominal pain such as mechanical small bowel obstruction, perforation of a hollow viscus, or appendicitis with fecalith. That said, the single-most important diagnostic test is arteriography, which can generally differentiate embolic from thrombotic occlusions. Emboli to the SMA usually lodge just proximal or distal to the origin of the middle colic artery. Thrombotic occlusions of preexistent stenotic lesions more often occur at the SMA origin and are associated with both generalized atherosclerosis of the aorta and the presence of extensive collaterals.

All patients with suspected embolic or thrombotic occlusions should undergo urgent laparotomy. Fluid resuscitation and administration of both heparin and antibiotics are indicated before surgery.

Chronic Mesenteric Ischemic Syndromes

Chronic mesenteric ischemia is most frequently associated with atherosclerotic occlusions or stenoses. Because of the abundant collateral network, multiple vessel involvement is usually required before classic postprandial symptoms occur. The presentation of chronic ischemia depends on the region of the gut affected. The most common syndromes involve the midgut (jejunum, ileum, and right colon) and reflect vascular insufficiency of the distribution of the SMA caused by atherosclerosis or midaortic developmental abnormalities. Because consumption of a meal predictably induces severe incapacitating pain, eating is dramatically curtailed ("food fear") and patients invariably lose weight. Weight loss is usually substantial and may exceed 25% of body mass.

Ischemia of the foregut (stomach and liver) is much less common and may be irregular in its symptomatology. Patients frequently describe nonspecific symptoms such as bloating and early satiety; food fear and weight loss are often absent.

Finally, ischemia of the hindgut (left colon and rectum) rarely presents with postprandial pain or weight loss. Patients present with hemoccult-positive diarrhea and chronic strictures caused by mucosal ischemia. These syndromes reflect insufficiency of the inferior mesenteric artery distribution usually because of atherosclerosis of the origin of the vessel associated with disease of the internal iliac arteries. Colonic ischemia may infrequently follow vascular reconstructions of the infrarenal aorta, which may inadvertently compromise collateral blood flow.

The definitive diagnosis of chronic intestinal ischemia is based on several factors, including: (1) symptoms consistent with the arterial obstructions; (2) exclusion of the other gastrointestinal pathology; and (3) arteriographic demonstration of appropriate occlusive lesions and collateral development. Selective arterial catheterizations are usually required together with oblique or lateral views to adequately image the origins of the three main visceral vessels. Recently, angioplasty with stent placement has been shown to be effective in treating these lesions. This approach is most attractive in higher-risk patients with severe malnutrition and hypoalbumenemia or limiting cardiac reserve. While initial relief of symptoms is very acceptable, sustained success is approximately 60 percent at 3 years in comparison with 80 percent in patients treated operatively. Vascular reconstruction for chronic foregut and midgut ischemia can be accomplished by endarterectomy or aortomesenteric bypass. In our practice, antegrade bypasses from the supraceliac aorta to the celiac axis and SMA are currently the most frequently used techniques and are described in detail in this chapter.

Patients with acute intestinal ischemia caused by embolus or thrombosis of the superior mesenteric artery usually present with the sudden onset of severe abdominal pain out of proportion to the patients' physical findings. The diagnosis must be made promptly and confirmed with arteriography so that surgery and revascularization can be carried out before bowel infarction occurs. Surgical exposure is obtained through a vertical midline incision, allowing thorough abdominal exploration and determination of intestinal viability.

The omentum and transverse colon are retracted superiorly, and the small bowel and mesentery are lifted and gently retracted to the patient's right. The superior mesenteric artery (SMA) is identified at the junction of the small bowel mesentery and transverse mesocolon as it crosses the duodenum. The peritoneum covering the mesentery is incised, and the SMA is gently dissected taking care to avoid injury to the superior mesenteric vein (SMV).

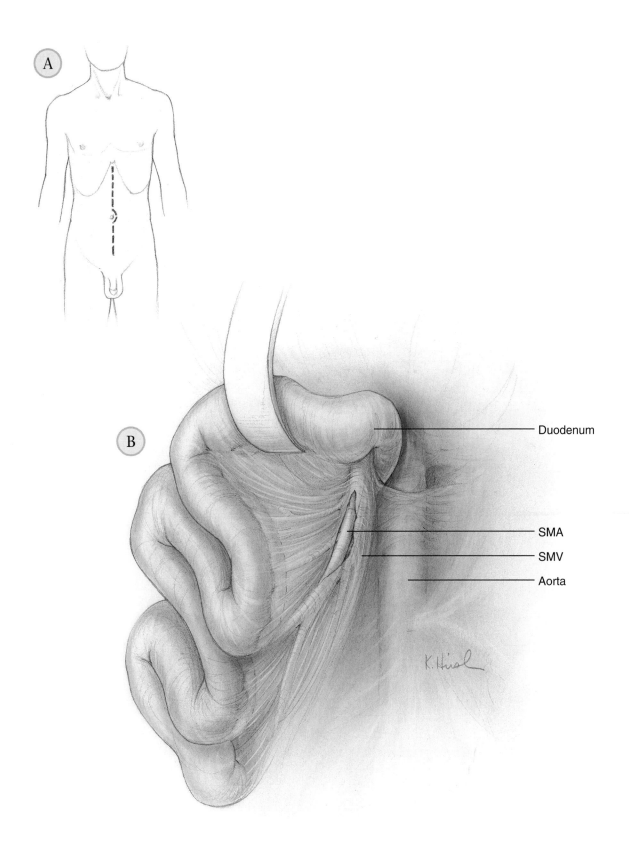

Duodenum

SMA

SMV

Aorta

The superior mesenteric artery is encircled with silastic tapes. After systemic heparinization, a transverse arteriotomy is performed and a balloon embolectomy catheter is gently advanced proximally, inflated, and withdrawn to remove the thromboembolus. The catheter is then passed distally to extract distal thrombus. If the clinical history and nature of the clot is consistent with embolus rather than *in situ* thrombosis of an occlusive lesion and excellent pulsatile inflow is obtained, bypass of the superior mesenteric artery may not be necessary.

The transverse arteriotomy may be closed with precise interrupted sutures.

If the artery is small, a vein patch may be necessary to avoid narrowing of the lumen.

After restoration of blood flow in the superior mesenteric artery, the bowel is carefully inspected to determine viability. Pulsations in the mesentery, the return of colon and peristalsis, and the presence of Doppler ultrasound signals on the antimesenteric border of the intestine are signs of intestinal viability. However, the gross visual appearance of the bowel after revascularization does not always guarantee long-term viability. The surgeon may wish to consider a second look operation after 24 hours to confirm intestinal viability.

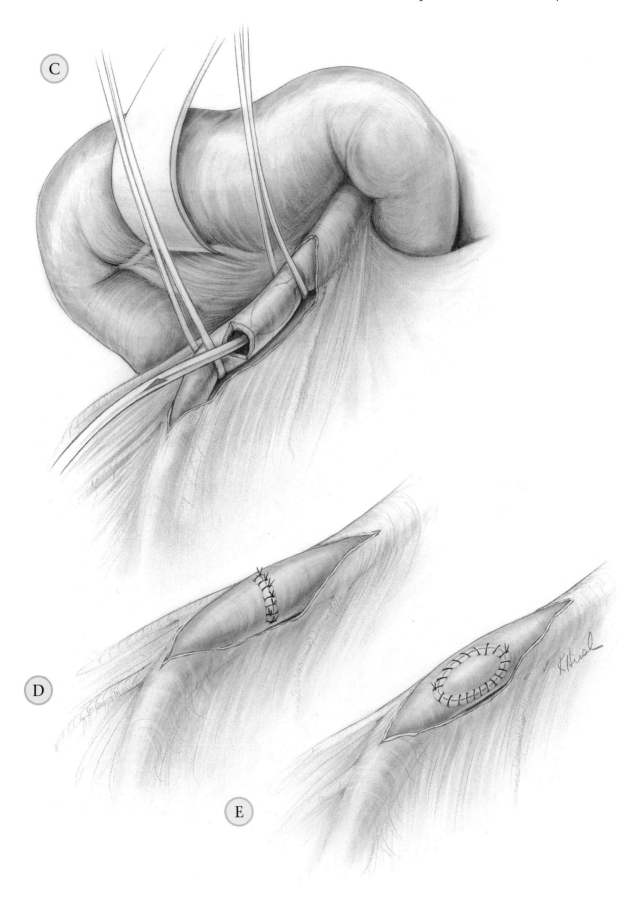

Patients with acute intestinal ischemia caused by thrombosis of preexistent occlusive lesions cannot be treated successfully with embolectomy techniques and require bypass procedures to revascularize the superior mesenteric artery. In the absence of intestinal perforation or infarction, prosthetic material may be used. However, if bowel infarction is present or contamination occurs during the procedure, saphenous vein must be used to avoid graft infection.

Patients with chronic mesenteric ischemia (visceral angina) present with postprandial abdominal pain and weight loss. Careful preoperative angiography is needed to properly demonstrate the celiac, superior mesenteric, and inferior mesenteric arteries and to plan visceral revascularization. We prefer to revascularize both the celiac and superior mesenteric arteries if both vessels are occluded.

A Aortosuperior mesenteric artery bypasses are useful in patients with acute mesenteric ischemia and in whom superior mesenteric embolectomy/thrombectomy has been unsuccessful in restoring blood flow. A reversed saphenous vein may be sutured end-to-side to the superior mesenteric artery at the site of the arteriotomy used for the embolectomy. This anastomosis is performed using 6–0 continuous monofilament suture. The graft is anastomosed to the aorta at a location that provides a satisfactory lie of the graft without kinking.

B Proper length of the saphenous vein bypass and location of the aortic anastomosis are critical in avoiding kinking of the graft when the small bowel mesentery is returned to the abdomen. The tendency of grafts in this location to kink limits the usefulness of anastomoses to the infrarenal aorta.

C Revascularization of the celiac axis can be accomplished using a bypass from the infrarenal aorta to a branch of the celiac axis such as the common hepatic artery. The right colon and duodenum are mobilized to the left past the inferior vena cava to expose the infrarenal abdominal aorta. The common hepatic artery is identified in the portal triad and dissected free. A saphenous vein or prosthetic bypass is sutured end-to-side to the infrarenal aorta. The bypass is passed retrograde behind the duodenum and head of the pancreas and anastomosed end-to-side to the hepatic artery using 6–0 monofilament suture. SMA, Superior mesenteric artery; SMV, superior mesenteric vein.

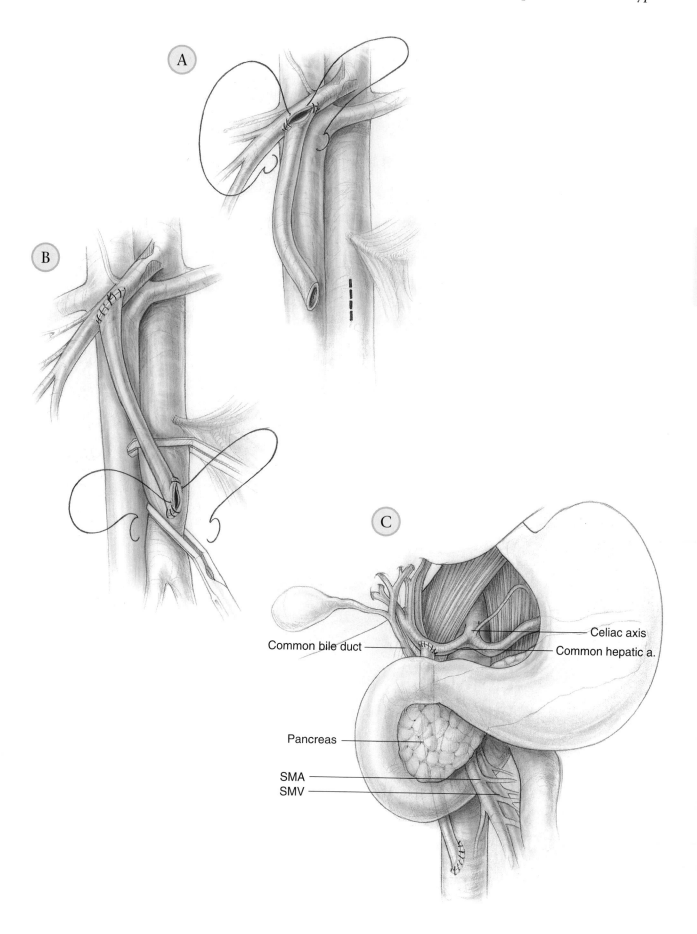

Common bile duct

Celiac axis

Common hepatic a.

Pancreas

SMA

SMV

Excellent operative exposure is afforded through an upper midline incision. Most patients requiring revascularization are thin or even emaciated.

After entering the "lesser space" through the gastrohepatic omentum, the left lobe of the liver is carefully reflected laterally with care to avoid injury to the hepatic veins.

The esophagus is identified after placement of a large nasogastric tube or bougé. The diaphragmatic crus is divided layer by layer using electrocautery, exposing the dense periarterial tissue of the celiac plexus. The supraceliac aorta and the entire celiac trunk are exposed.

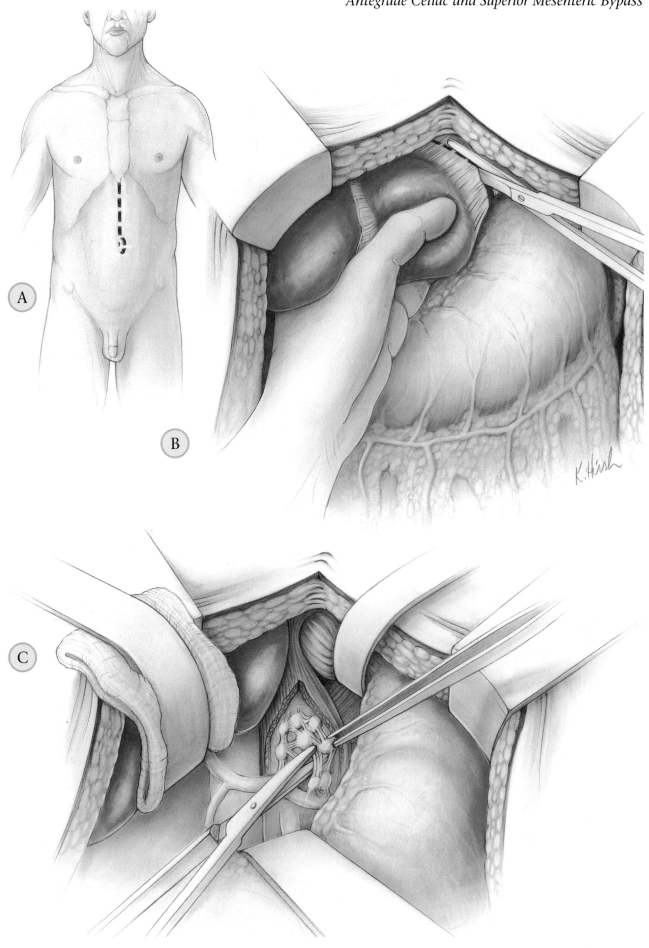

After heparinization and reduction in systemic systolic blood pressure to 90–110 mm Hg, aortic occlusion is obtained by placement of a partially occlusive Lemole clamp (as shown) or two aortic clamps above and below the supraceliac segment. In the technique illustrated, a single-graft limb is anastomosed to the aorta with a 3–0 monofilament suture. A suitable opening is made in the graft, allowing for end-to-side anastomosis of the cut end of the main celiac trunk. After the proximal clamp removal, the graft is then passed behind the pancreas and to the left of the aorta in a tunnel previously created using blunt finger dissection. An end-to-side anastomosis is performed to the SMA distal to the occlusive lesion (not shown).

An alternative reconstruction employs similar intraoperative exposure, but utilizes a bifurcated 12 × 6 graft. The limbs are then anastomosed to the celiac artery end-to-end, and the superior mesenteric artery end-to-side. Note the direct route of both graft limbs, which minimizes kinking.

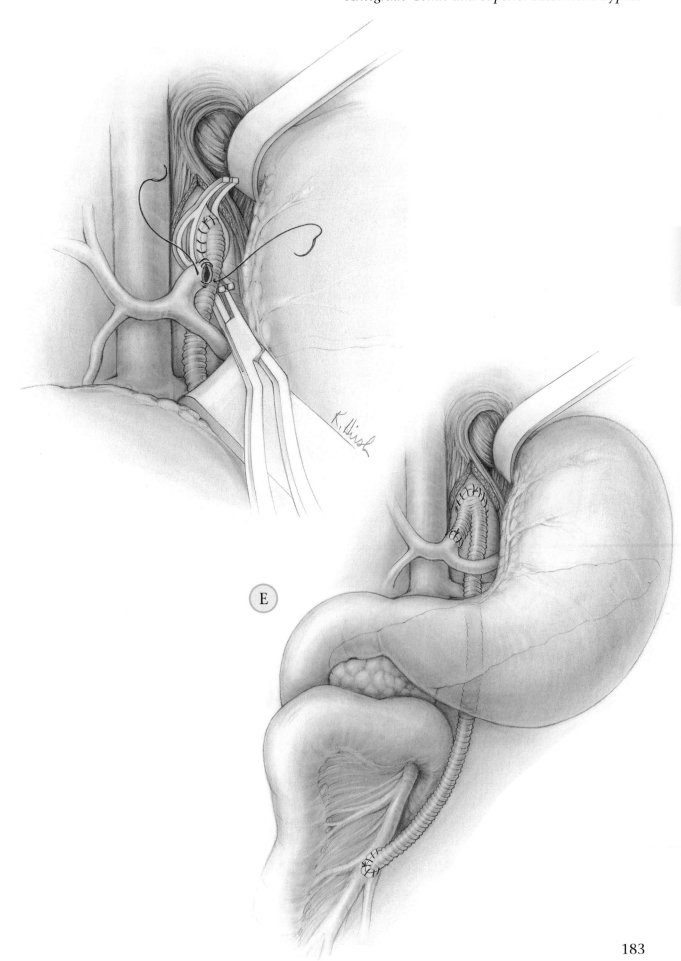

Orifice occlusive lesions involving both the celiac and superior mesenteric arteries are usually best endarterectomized through a transaortic approach. This approach has the advantage of removing atheroma from the aorta and visceral branch orifices during the same procedure. This may be accomplished through a transperitoneal or retroperitoneal approach to the perivisceral aorta. This section will demonstrate the midline transperitoneal medial visceral approach. The retroperitoneal exposure to the perivisceral aorta is shown on pp. 79–81.

A   A generous midline incision is made allowing adequate exposure of the entire upper abdominal aorta.

B   An incision is made along the retroperitoneum, posterior to the left colon and spleen, to allow atraumatic medial visceral rotation.

C   Continuous exposure of the aorta and the celiac axis, superior mesenteric artery, and inferior mesenteric artery can be gained.

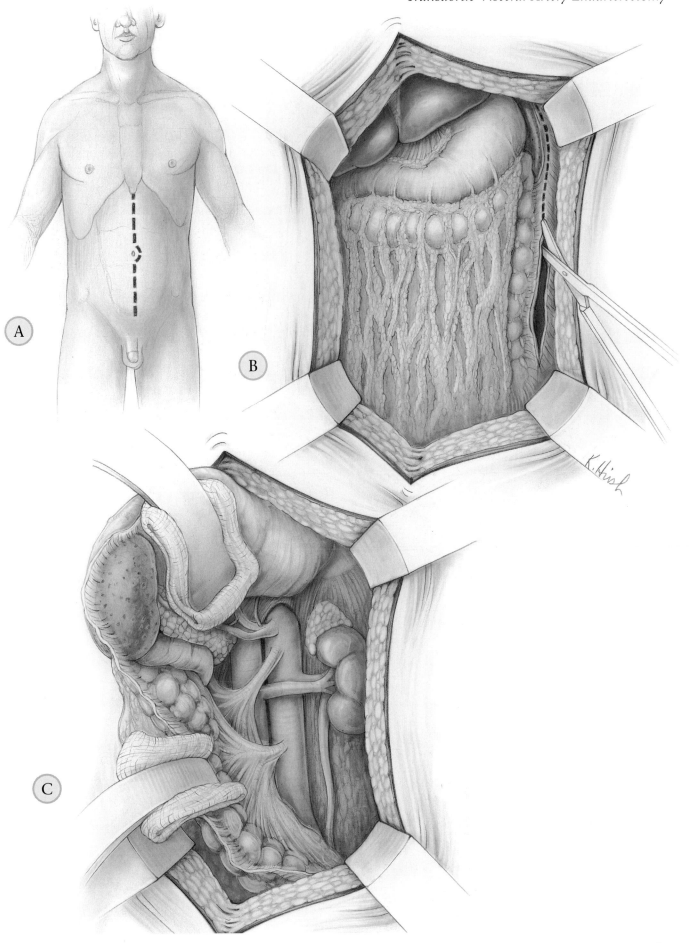

The spleen, pancreas, stomach, and colon are reflected anterior and medial exposing the origins of the celiac and superior mesenteric arteries.

After dissection and control of both renal arteries, an arteriotomy is made in the aorta anterior to the left renal artery. The incision is continued superiorly above the celiac axis. Transverse arteriotomies that fashion a "trap door" incision are then made in the aorta. SMA, Superior mesenteric artery.

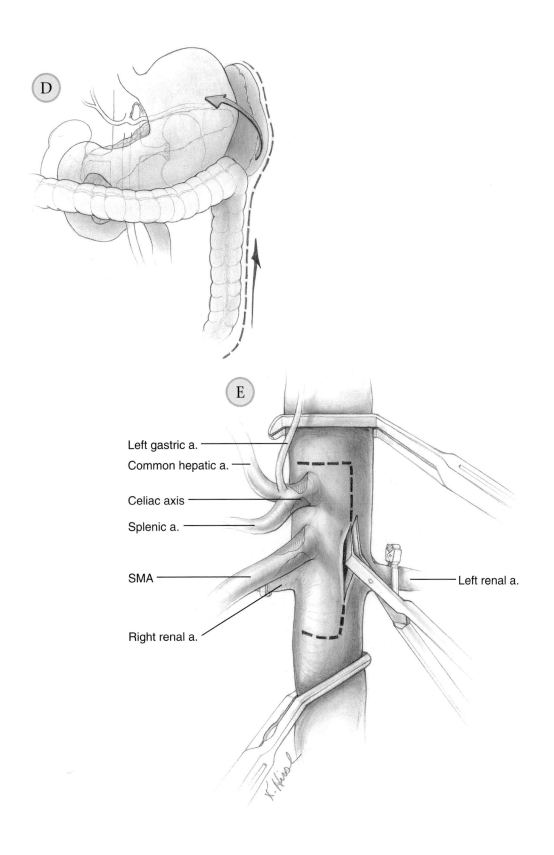

The aortic atheroma is removed. Plaque extensions into the orifices of the celiac artery, superior mesenteric artery, and both renal arteries are removed by eversion technique. If satisfactory distal end points are not obtained on all vessels, the distal end point must be exposed and intimal tacking sutures placed to avoid postoperative thrombosis.

The arteriotomy is closed with continuous 4–0 monofilament suture. Distal blood flow in all four vessels should be critically assessed by palpation and Doppler examination. Any abnormalities must be evaluated by intraoperative angiogram. This can be performed by clamping the aorta above the celiac axis and below the renal arteries and injecting contrast into the isolated aortic segment, or selective transfemoral intraoperative arteriography.

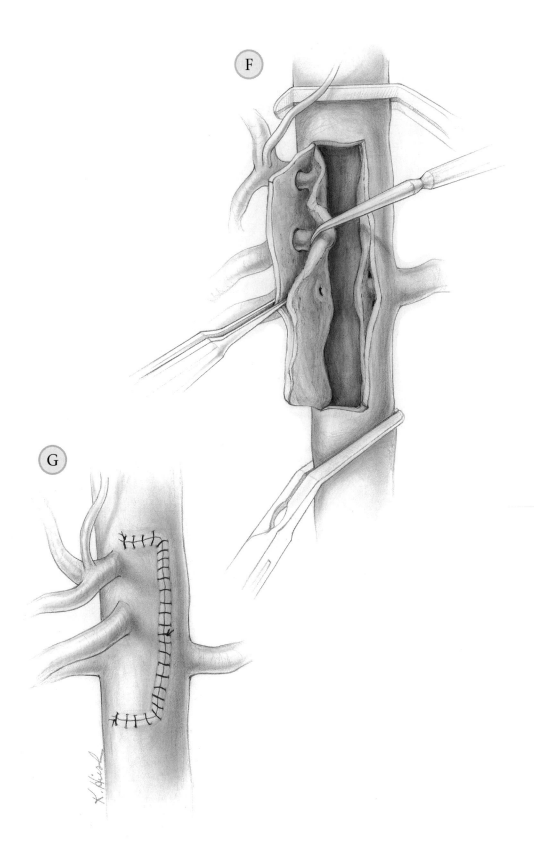

(A) If occlusive lesions involve only the proximal superior mesenteric artery, a localized endarterectomy may be performed.

(B) After proximal and distal control of the aorta, a longitudinal arteriotomy is made in the superior mesenteric artery and carried down into the aorta.

(C) An endarterectomy is performed with care being taken to obtain a satisfactory distal end point in the superior mesenteric artery.

(D) A prosthetic or vein graft patch is placed over the arteriotomy using continuous suture technique.

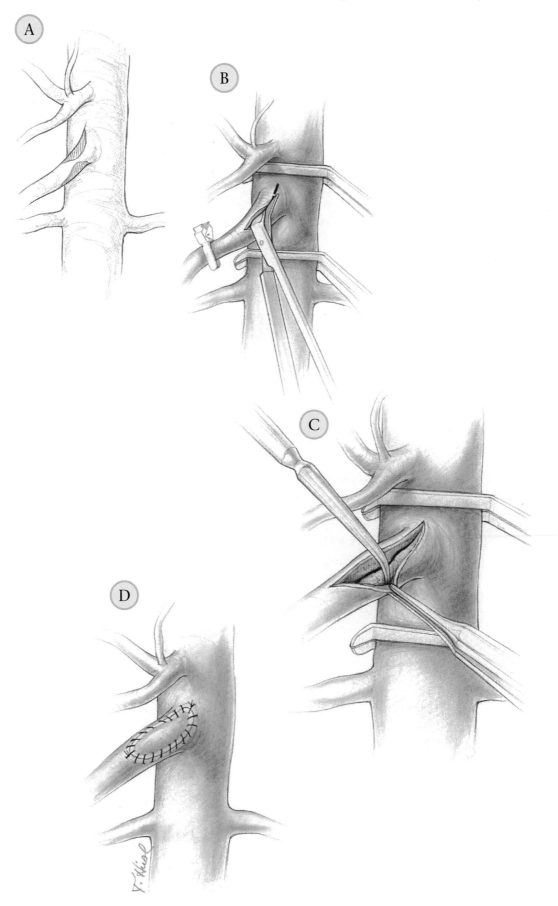

SECTION V

Peripheral Occlusive Disease

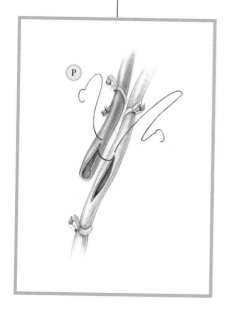

The progressive manifestations of peripheral arterial occlusive disease of the lower extremities are intermittent claudication, rest pain, skin ulceration, and gangrene. Intermittent claudication is a syndrome of pain or fatigue in large muscle groups that occurs with exercise and is relieved by rest. It can be distinguished from other causes of leg pain by the absence of pain at initiation of movement and the reproducibility of symptoms after specific intervals of walking. It is characteristic that the level of claudication is generally one anatomic level below the point of arterial obstruction. Aortoiliac occlusive disease leads to claudication in the hips and buttocks, as well as impotence; superficial femoral artery obstruction commonly causes calf claudication alone. The natural history of claudication is generally benign with only a 5% risk for gangrene within 5 years if treated conservatively. Nonetheless, the effect of severe claudication on the quality of life is often considerable.

The presence of rest pain indicates a much more severe degree of ischemia. Typically, patients experience pain in the toes and head of the metatarsals because of inadequate neural blood supply. This chronic debilitating pain is most evident during the night and commonly causes patients to awaken from sleep. Temporary relief is obtained by dangling the affected leg over the side of the bed or getting up and walking. The outlook for patients with rest pain is far worse than that for patients with claudication. If left untreated, nearly 50% of patients with rest pain require amputation for intractable pain or gangrene within 2 years.

The most advanced manifestations of severe arterial insufficiency are cutaneous ulcers and gangrene. Although the underlying cause of these lesions is severe ischemia from arterial occlusive disease, the inciting event is often minor skin trauma. The ischemic arterial ulcer is most commonly found on the toes, heel, dorsum of the foot, or lower third of the leg. The pain is severe, persistent, and worsens at night. The ulcer itself is generally "punched out" with a pale or necrotic base.

The final stage of arterial insufficiency is gangrene. Dry gangrene refers to mummification of tissue without purulence or cellulites. In this chronic ischemic state, relatively insignificant volumes of bacteria can overcome local defense mechanisms and progress rapidly to limb and life-threatening infections (wet gangrene). The latter condition is an indication for aggressive treatment to prevent ascending infection. This includes urgent debridement of the infected tissue, high doses of appropriate antibiotics, and prompt revascularization of the extremity.

The diagnosis of peripheral vascular occlusive disease can usually be established by a careful history and physical examination. In addition to the absence of distal pulses and the symptoms described earlier, more subtle physical findings include loss of hair on the extremities, thinning of the skin, and atrophy of the distal musculature.

Noninvasive tests including Doppler-derived pressure measurements and velocity waveforms can aid in determining the level and severity of disease. Findings consistent with aortoiliac disease include diminished high-thigh arterial pressures and monophasic or biphasic velocity waveforms at the femoral level. Substantial decreases in ankle–brachial indices with exercise may also suggest aortoiliac disease.

The indications for invasive therapy are limited to incapacitating claudication, rest pain, and threatened loss of limb manifest by ulceration and gangrene. In the latter two categories, the decision to proceed with operation, angioplasty, or both is easily justified. The proper management of patients with claudication is more difficult. Before any form of invasive treatment, both patient and physician should be convinced that exercise-related reports substantially interfere with employment or lifestyle.

If patients have limb-threatening conditions or incapacitating claudication, angioplasty or operative treatment is appropriate. Transluminal balloon angioplasty offers the advantages of a low incidence of serious complications, minimal hospitalization, and little, if any, postprocedural restrictions of activity. Angioplasty is most successful in treatment of isolated hemodynamically significant lesions of the iliac or superficial femoral arteries with severe symptoms. Other favorable clinical situations include stenoses of previously placed bypass grafts.

Results from angioplasty depend on a multiplicity of factors including the nature of the lesion (stenosis vs. occlusion), the site dilated, and the length of the stenosis. In the iliac region, more than 90% of lesions can be successfully dilated with a 70% 2-year patency. Angioplasty of the superficial femoral arteries has less impressive results. Initial success rates of 75% decrease to approximately 50% at 2 years, depending on patient selection.

Bypass procedures as described in this section are the standard operative treatments for lower extremity peripheral occlusive disease. For discussion purposes, bypasses can be divided into "inflow" (suprainguinal) and "outflow" (infrainguinal) procedures.

The most common surgical procedure for aortoiliac obstructions is the aorto-bifemoral bypass graft. In this operation, a prosthetic graft is sutured to the infrarenal aorta proximally and the common femoral arteries distally. In the presence of a superficial femoral artery obstruction, the profunda artery can be used as the primary outflow bed. Aortofemoral bypass grafting is a stable and durable operation; the 5-year patency rate is greater than 90%, and perioperative mortality is low (about 3%). When such operations are not successful, these failures are impacted by the presence of coronary artery disease, which is endemic to this patient population.

Patients who require bypass of an aortoiliac lesion, but are too ill to withstand an aortobifemoral graft, may be treated by subcutaneous axillofemoral or femoro-femoral bypass grafts. Unfortunately, these grafts fail more frequently than aorto-bifemoral grafts because of their longer length (implying increased resistance) and the risk for external compression in subcutaneous tunnels. For this reason, extraanatomic grafts should be considered only when aortofemoral grafts or local endarterectomies are not feasible.

"Outflow procedures" include all bypasses of the infrainguinal vessels (femoropopliteal or femorotibial bypasses). Autogenous saphenous vein (either reversed or *in situ*) is the best conduit for such procedures. If the saphenous vein has been used for another procedure or is not suitable for bypass, then prosthetic materials can be inserted. These prosthetic materials do not have the longevity of the saphenous vein but have acceptable results.

Limb salvage rates for these procedures at 5 years are about 75% for femoropopliteal bypass grafts and 50% for femoral tibial bypass grafts. Limb salvage rates are usually 15% greater than the patency rates of the grafts. The long-term success of each bypass graft depends on the inflow, the type of conduit used, the outflow bed, and the technical aspects of the procedure. Thrombosis is the most serious early complication and is usually caused by technical error or inadequate outflow for the graft. Prompt thrombectomy or, in selected cases, local thrombolysis and recognition of any underlying technical problems will usually restore patency of the graft.

Aortofemoral bypass requires surgical exposure of the infrarenal aorta and both common femoral arteries. The arteries may be exposed through a transperitoneal or retroperitoneal approach. The retroperitoneal approach is particularly useful in patients who have had previous intraabdominal surgery, and those with colostomies, marked obesity, or pulmonary compromise. The transperitoneal approach is more familiar to most surgeons and permits assessment of other intraabdominal organs. We favor the retroperitoneal approach for most cases, because exposure is excellent, perioperative fluid requirements are lessened, and small bowel function frequently returns earlier.

(A) The transperitoneal approach to the abdominal aorta can be made through either a vertical midline abdominal incision or a transverse infraumbilical incision. Vertical incisions are made over the common femoral arteries below the inguinal ligament.

(B) After exploration of the intraabdominal organs, the transverse colon is retracted superiorly and the small bowel is displaced to the right. The use of a plastic bowel bag for the small bowel and packing the transverse colon within the abdomen in the superior portion of the wound minimize evaporative water loss during the procedure. The sigmoid colon is packed off in the left lower quadrant. An incision is made in the parietal peritoneum overlying the aorta and extended up to include the ligament of Treitz. The fourth portion of the duodenum is mobilized and retracted to the right to expose the left renal vein as it crosses over the abdominal aorta. The left renal vein is a useful landmark, for it identifies the level of the renal arteries, which lies behind and slightly superior to the level of the renal vein. Mobilization of the left renal vein protects it from injury and facilitates dissection of the infrarenal segment of abdominal aorta.

Aortofemoral bypass grafts should be placed in the proximal portion of the infrarenal aorta 2 to 3 cm below the renal arteries. More distal anastomotic sites should be avoided to prevent the possibility of later graft compromise by progression of atherosclerosis in the proximal infrarenal aorta. A limited segment of aorta needs to be exposed between the renal arteries and the inferior mesenteric artery (IMA). It is not necessary to expose the aorta below the IMA, and dissection of the aortic bifurcation should be avoided to minimize risk for postoperative neurogenic erectile dysfunction. The groin incisions are made directly over the common femoral arteries, which are exposed from the inguinal ligament to their bifurcation into the superficial femoral and profunda femoris arteries. Individual control of the superficial femoral and profunda femoral vessels is obtained. Branches of the profunda femoris vein cross over the first portion of the profunda femoris artery and may need to be divided to facilitate exposure of the profunda. The posterior portion of the inguinal ligament should be divided along with the fascia of the transversus abdominus muscle, as it crosses the femoral artery, to provide adequate space for tunnelling of the graft. This tunnel should easily admit one to two fingers to avoid graft compression. During tunnelling, care should be exercised to avoid circumflex femoral veins that can cross the external iliac artery underneath the inguinal ligament.

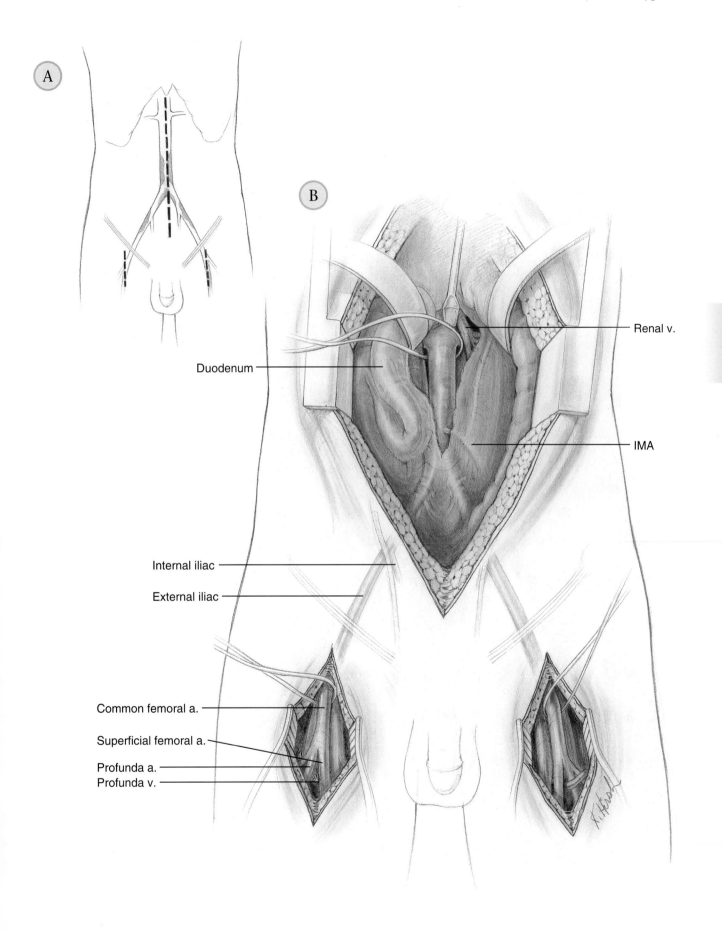

For the retroperitoneal approach to the abdominal aorta, the patient is positioned on a bean bag with shoulders at a 45-degree angle and the left arm supported on a sling anteriorly and superiorly. The pelvis should be as flat as possible. An incision is made in the left flank extending from two fingerbreadths below the umbilicus to the tip of the twelfth rib. The external and internal oblique muscles are divided, and the left rectus muscle is divided. The transversus abdominus muscle fibers are split. The peritoneum, which lies immediately below the transversus abdominus muscle, is carefully separated from the muscle laterally and from the posterior rectus sheath medially. The peritoneum is mobilized superiorly to the costal cartilages and inferiorly to the anterior superior iliac spine.

The peritoneum is retracted to the right until the iliopsoas muscle and ureter are visible. The plane between the left colon anteriorly and the ureter posteriorly is then developed, mobilizing the colon to the right and leaving the kidney and ureter posteriorly. The left renal vein is visualized as it crosses the aorta and identifies the level of the infrarenal aorta required for anastomosis.

Alternatively, it is possible to approach the aorta in a plane behind the kidney. Gerota's capsule surrounding the kidney is mobilized together with the peritoneum. In this exposure, the ureter and gonadal vein will not be seen, but the left renal artery will be identified from behind. Either approach will give satisfactory exposure of the infrarenal aorta. A variety of self-retaining retractors are useful for maintaining exposure of the aorta during the procedure. IMA, Inferior mesenteric artery; IVC, inferior vena cava.

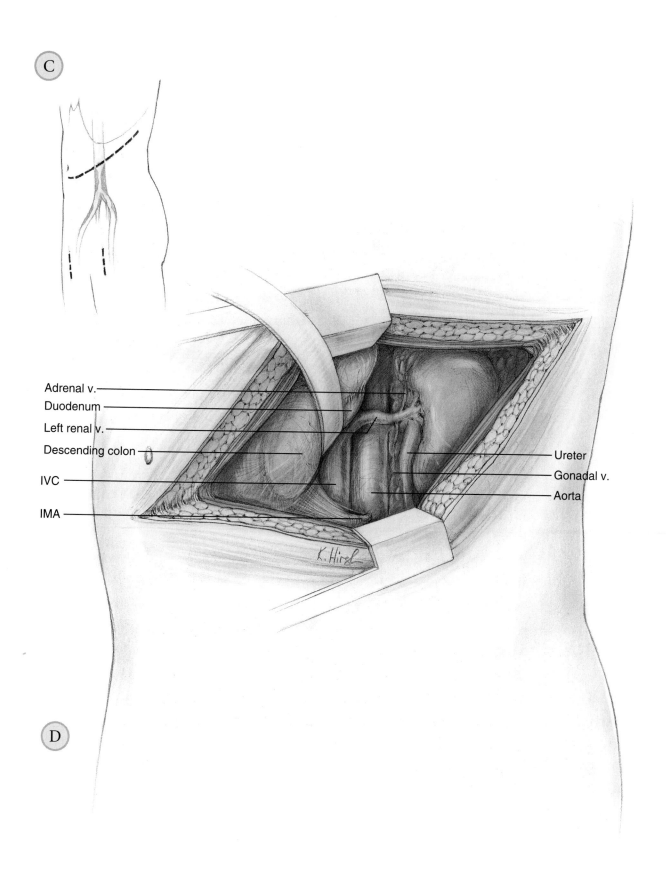

Adrenal v.

Duodenum

Left renal v.

Descending colon

IVC

IMA

Ureter

Gonadal v.

Aorta

K. Hirel

C

D

(E) A suitably sized Dacron bifurcation graft is selected based on the size of the infrarenal aorta. Most commonly, this is a 16 × 8 mm bifurcation graft. A variety of graft materials including woven Dacron, knitted Dacron, and polytetrafluoroethylene are available. We most commonly perform end-to-end anastomoses because of superior hemodynamic configuration. However, under certain circumstances end-to-side anastomoses are advisable (see Figs. A, B, C, page 213). After systemic heparinization (100 mg/kg), the infrarenal aorta is cross-clamped just below the renal arteries. The infrarenal aorta is transected.

(F) The distal aortic stump is oversewn with continuous 3–0 nonabsorbable monofilament suture. Deep sutures are placed. Two rows of suture may be required for a secure closure. If extensive calcific plaque is encountered, a local endarterectomy may be required to allow closure.

(G) The proximal aortic stump is inspected. Thrombus material or loose irregular intimal plaque is removed. However, care must be exercised and an extensive deep endarterectomy should be avoided or the aortic wall will become too thin to hold sutures.

(H) The prosthetic bypass is then sutured end-to-end to the infrarenal aorta using 3–0 continuous monofilament nonabsorbable suture. Large "bites" of the aorta should be taken and care must be exercised to follow the curve of the needle so that longitudinal tears in the aorta are not produced during suture placement. Sutures should not be placed too close together to avoid concentrating needle holes and tension in one area of the vessel. One continuous suture, beginning posteriorly, extending around to the sides, and tied anteriorly, is usually sufficient.

After completion of the suture line, the Dacron graft is pinched shut with the left hand, and the infrarenal aortic clamp is slowly released with the right hand to check the proximal suture line. Any defects in the aortic suture line should be repaired at this time with additional sutures. If longitudinal tears in the aorta are present, these should be repaired with fine pledgeted sutures. The graft is checked at this time by allowing the body of the graft to fill with blood. Minor oozing through the interstices of the graft will seal in several minutes by intermittently filling the graft with blood, even with the patient fully heparinized. After verifying that the proximal anastomosis is satisfactory, the graft should be emptied of blood and flushed with heparinized saline to prevent clot formation within the prosthesis during subsequent stages of the operation.

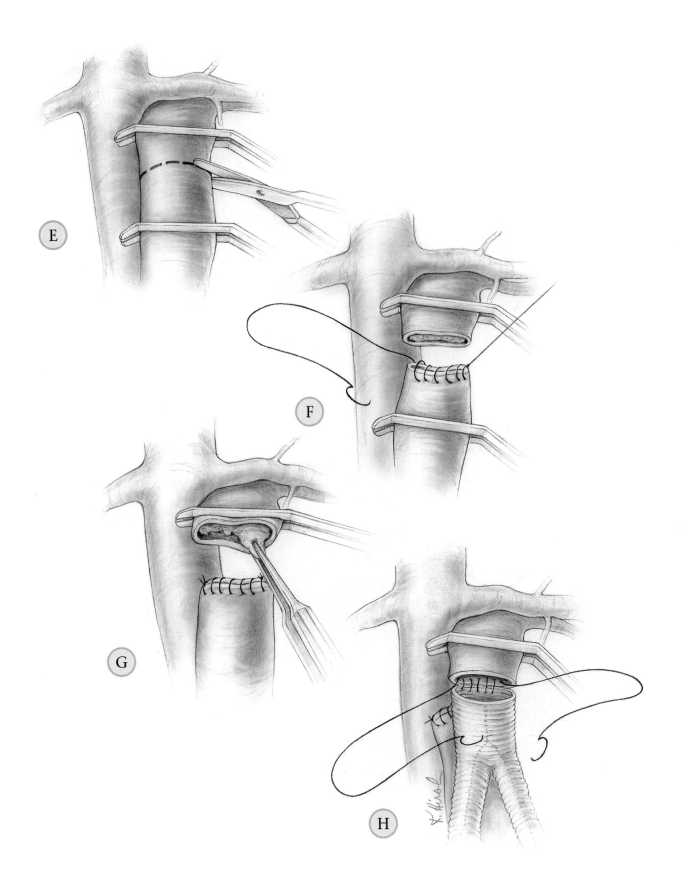

Ⓘ A tunnel is created from the aorta to the femoral artery along the course of the iliac artery. This is accomplished using blunt finger dissection. The ureter is swept anteriorly, and the iliac artery must be palpable immediately below the index finger along the entire length of the path from the aorta to the groin. A long, curved clamp is placed from the groin to touch the index finger in the tunnel and then gently guided along the course of the iliac artery to the level of the aorta.

Ⓙ The right limb of the graft is grasped by the clamp and gently delivered to the groin. A similar procedure is performed for the left limb of the graft, which is tunnelled along the course of the left iliac artery behind the left ureter to the groin. Great care must be exercised to ensure that the graft does not pass anterior to the ureter. If so, the ureter can be compressed between the rigid iliac artery posteriorly and the pulsatile Dacron graft anteriorly.

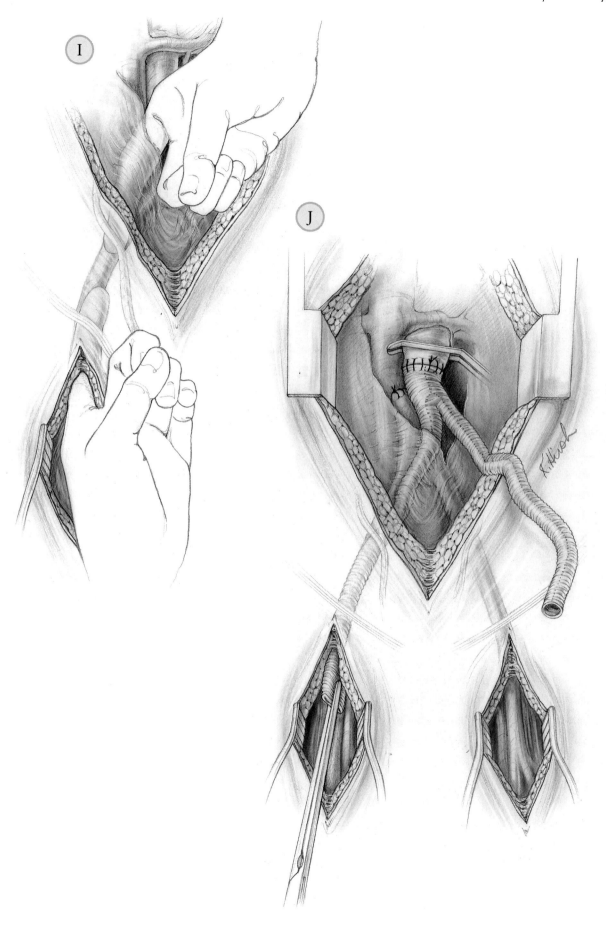

K   Vascular clamps are applied to the common femoral, superficial femoral, and profunda femoris arteries, and a longitudinal arteriotomy is made in the common femoral artery. If significant calcific or ulcerated plaque is present, a femoral endarterectomy may be necessary. If there is an orifice stenosis of either the superficial femoral or profunda femoris artery, the arteriotomy may need to be extended into one or both of the outflow vessels.

L   The Dacron graft is stretched and cut to suit the length of the anastomosis. A graft that is too long may buckle and kink, and a graft that is too short will produce excess tension on the suture line and may predispose to pseudoaneurysm formation. Proper length is best determined by pinching the end of the Dacron graft, releasing the proximal aortic clamp, and allowing the graft to fill at normal arterial pressure.

M   The anastomosis to the femoral artery is begun using 4–0 or 5–0 monofilament nonabsorbable suture. Continuous sutures are placed, securing the full thickness of the femoral artery. Great care must be exercised to carefully visualize each suture placement, particularly about the toe of the graft, to avoid intimal flaps or other technical defects.

N   The anastomosis of the aortofemoral bypass to the right femoral artery is completed, and preparations are made to unclamp the aorta and revascularize the right leg. Five to 10 minutes before reaching this stage in the operation the surgeon should notify the anesthesiologist that he will soon be unclamping the aorta. This will allow the anesthesiologist to ensure that the patient is properly hydrated so that "declamping hypotension" can be avoided.

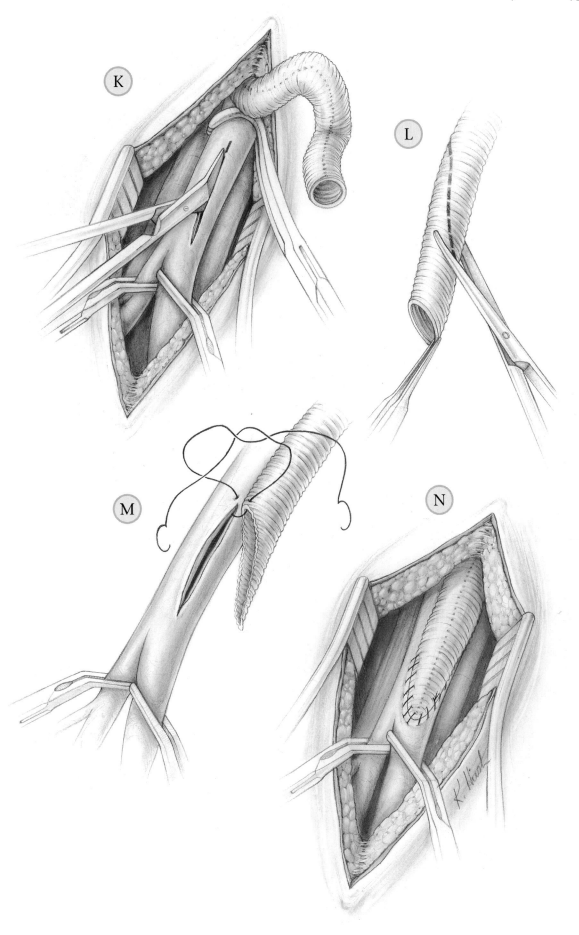

The distal clamps of the right groin are briefly released allowing back bleeding from the superficial femoral and profunda femoris vessels to fill the Dacron graft. This back bleeding removes air from the Dacron graft. The surgeon can confirm that all air has been evacuated by demonstrating free bleeding from the as yet unanastomosed left limb of the aortofemoral bypass graft.

After the right limb of the graft is filled with blood, it is occluded, and the proximal aortic clamp is released, allowing the force of blood flow to flush out the graft through the open left limb. This evacuates any thrombus or debris that may have collected at the proximal clamp during the procedure.

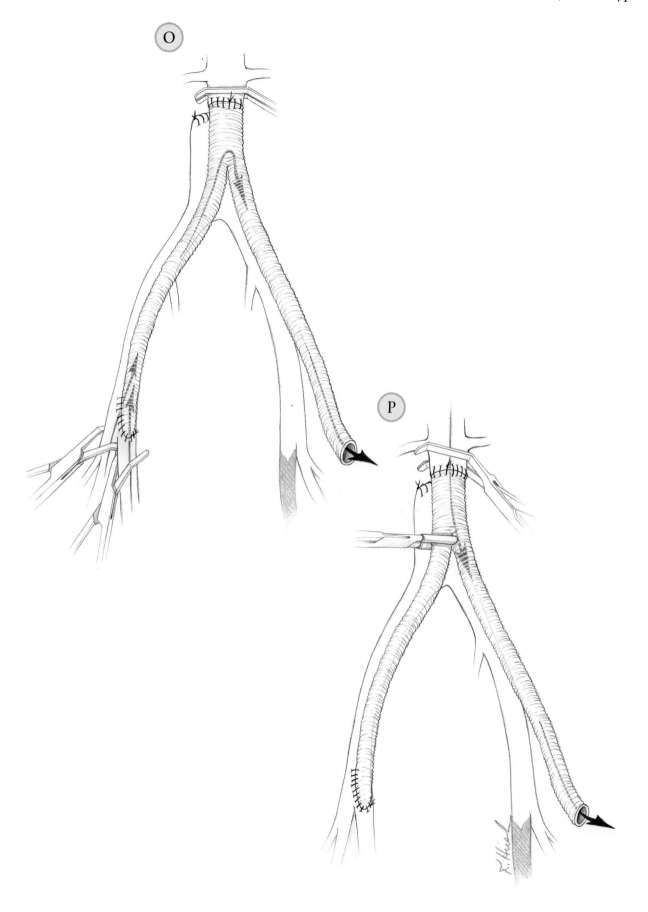

Q A rubbershod clamp is then placed on the left limb of the bypass graft. The superficial femoral and profunda clamps are reapplied and the proximal aortic clamp is released to allow blood flow into the right limb of the graft, exiting retrograde through the common femoral artery up the external iliac artery. Directing this first flow of blood in a retrograde fashion prevents distal embolization of thrombotic material into the right leg. After a few seconds, the superficial femoral and profunda clamps are removed and flow is restored to the right leg. Immediately after restoring flow to the leg, the surgeon should be in constant communication with the anesthesiologist and should monitor arterial pressures to detect "declamping hypotension." Should this occur, the surgeon can partially or totally obstruct the right limb of the graft between his fingers to increase outflow resistance, thereby increasing systemic arterial pressure. Should such maneuvers be necessary, the surgeon should intermittently allow one or two pulses to travel through the graft, because prolonged periods of stasis in a blood-filled graft may result in thrombus formation.

R The left limb of the graft should be evacuated of blood and rinsed with heparinized saline so that thrombus does not form in the left limb during the anastomosis to the left femoral artery. Clamps are applied to the femoral artery and its branches. In this instance, the superficial femoral artery is occluded; therefore, a clamp is not required. A Heifetz clamp is usually satisfactory for the profunda femoris artery. The arteriotomy begins in the common femoral artery and is extended into the profunda femoris artery, because the profunda is the only outflow for this limb of the graft. The profunda arteriotomy should be extended to whatever level is necessary to ensure that any proximal orifice lesion in the profunda has been bypassed.

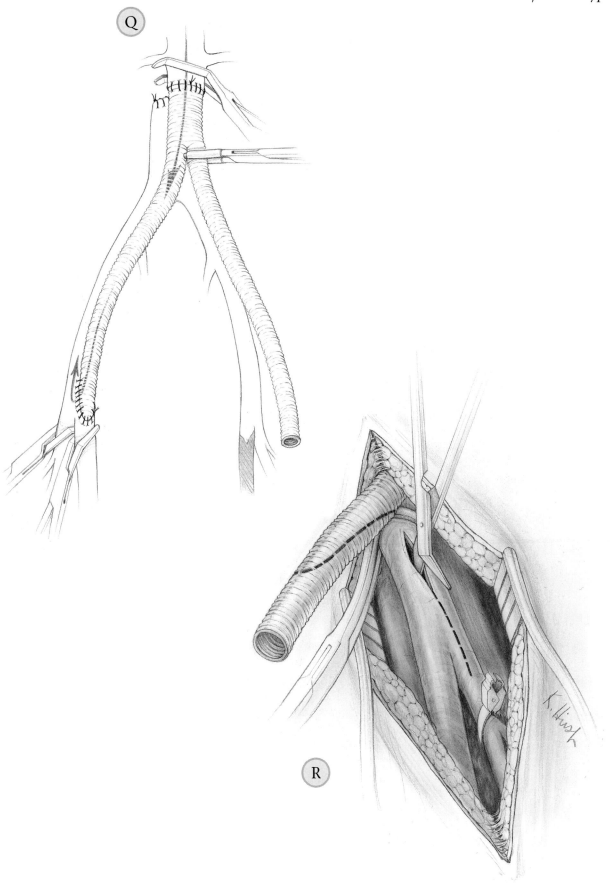

The anastomosis of the left limb of the graft is performed using 4–0 or 5–0 monofilament running suture. If the arteriotomy must be extended quite a distance on the profunda, 5–0 suture is preferred because of the fragile nature and thin wall of the profunda. Precise placement of the sutures is needed to avoid intimal flaps and irregularities.

Before completion of the anastomosis, the left limb of the bypass is flushed by releasing the proximal clamp to evacuate air, thrombus, and debris from the graft. The suture line is then completed, and flow is established through the left limb of the graft retrograde through the common femoral and external iliac arteries. The profunda clamp is then released and flow is restored to the left leg. The anesthesiologist should be notified of the imminent revascularization of the left limb, and care must be taken to avoid declamping hypotension.

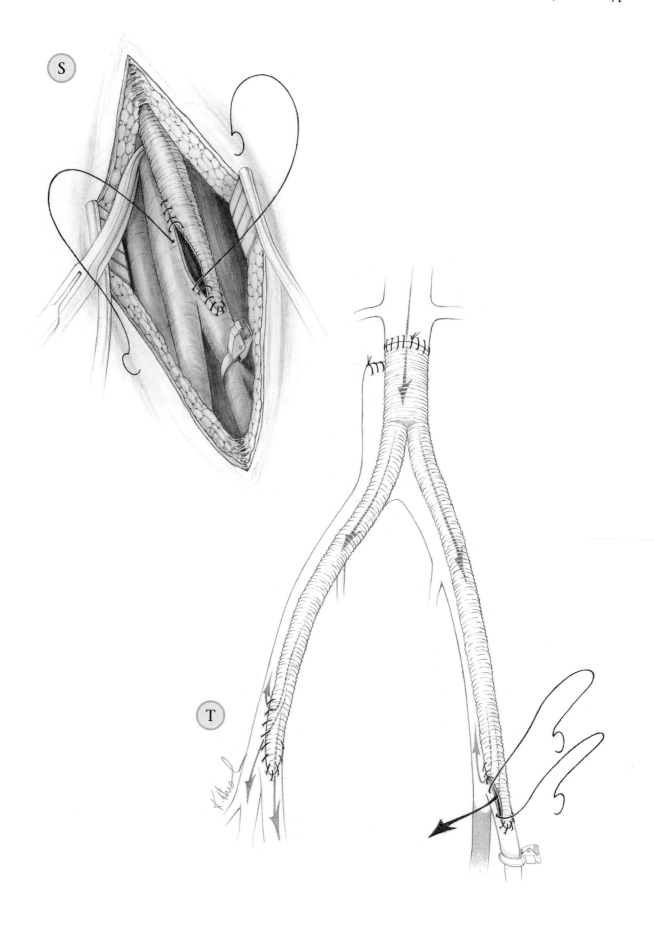

In instances where there is bilateral external iliac obstruction that precludes pelvic perfusion through retrograde flow from the femoral artery through the external iliac arteries, it is advisable to use an end-to-side proximal aortic anastomosis. An end-to-side proximal anastomosis will preserve flow through the distal aorta in an antegrade fashion and permit internal iliac and IMA perfusion.

The aorta is exposed as required in an end-to-end anastomosis. Instead of transecting the infrarenal aorta, a longitudinal arteriotomy is made. The aorta is inspected, and a local endarterectomy is performed if necessary. The aortic bifurcation graft is cut obliquely and matched to the size of the aortotomy. The graft is anastomosed to the aorta with continuous 3–0 monofilament nonabsorbable suture. Large, secure sutures are placed in the aorta.

After completion of the anastomosis, the aortic clamps are removed and a clamp is placed on the Dacron graft. The graft is tunnelled to the groins in the same fashion as in an end-to-end aortofemoral bypass graft. The duration of aortic clamping is less with end-to-side anastomosis, and declamping hypotension is unusual.

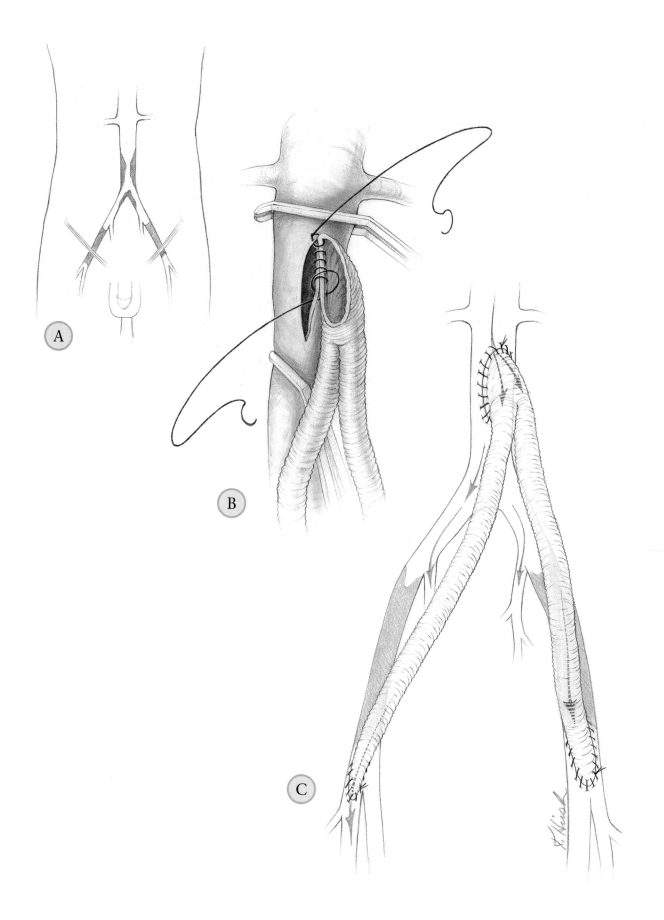

Axillofemoral bypass grafts are used as extraanatomic bypasses to revascularize the lower extremities in instances where standard aortofemoral or aortoiliac bypass grafts cannot be used. The usual indication is the need to revascularize the lower legs before or after removal of an infected aortic graft. Although the operation is usually called an axillofemoral bypass, in fact, the subclavian artery is the inflow vessel. The distal anastomosis is performed to the femoral artery in an area outside the infected field. This may require anastomosis to the common femoral, superficial femoral, or profunda femoral arteries.

A The patient is placed supine on the operating room table with the arm extended on an arm board. This positioning elevates the distal portion of the clavicle, allowing easy exposure of the subclavian artery. Either the right or left subclavian artery may be used as a donor vessel and the least diseased should be selected. In general, atherosclerotic lesions are more common in the proximal left subclavian artery than in the innominate or right subclavian artery. Blood pressures should be determined in both upper extremities before surgery, but angiography is usually not necessary. The handedness of a person may also influence the choice of a right- or left-sided graft. In the case illustrated, the patient has an infected aortoiliac bypass. Incisions are made in both groins for exposure of the common femoral arteries.

B An incision is made one fingerbreadth below the clavicle and runs from the level of the coracoid process to the sternoclavicular joint. The fibers of the pectoralis major muscle are split, and the cephalic vein may be seen penetrating the clavipectoral fascia to join the subclavian vein. The clavipectoral fascia is divided, and the subclavian vein is exposed.

C The subclavian vein is mobilized and retracted inferiorly, and the subclavian artery is exposed just distal to its exit from the thoracic outlet. The pectoralis minor muscle may sometimes be seen laterally, but if this muscle is a prominent part of the operative field, the surgical exposure is too far lateral. The highest thoracic artery can be seen originating in the proximal portion of the subclavian artery. This branch is divided to permit complete mobilization of the proximal portion of the subclavian artery.

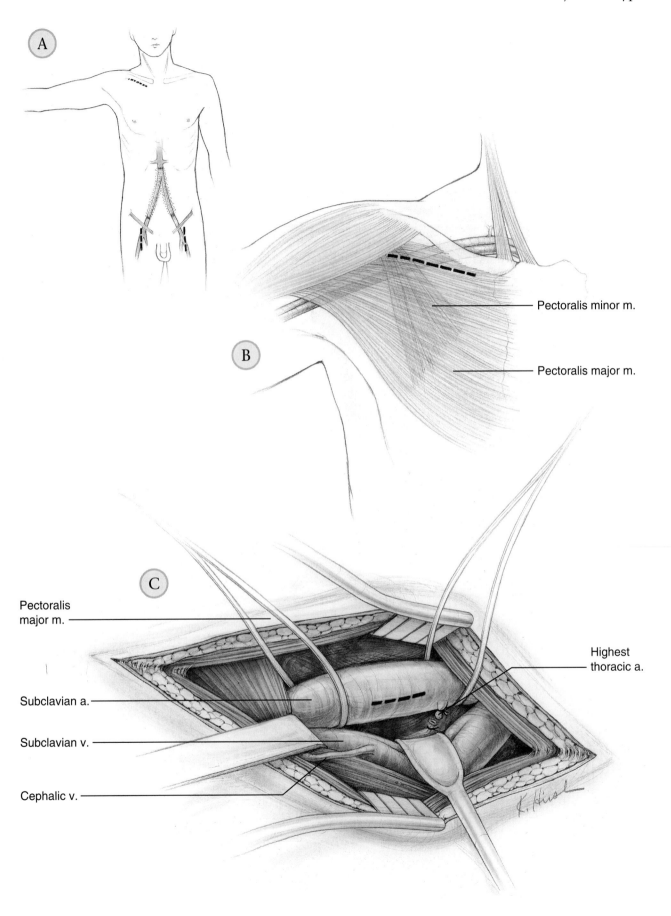

Pectoralis minor m.

Pectoralis major m.

Pectoralis major m.

Highest thoracic a.

Subclavian a.

Subclavian v.

Cephalic v.

After exposure of the common femoral, superficial femoral, and profunda femoral vessels, a tunnel is created between the subclavian artery and femoral artery using a long tunnelling instrument. This is passed along the chest wall deep to the pectoralis minor muscle. It then runs along the midaxillary line in a subcutaneous plane, crosses anterior to the anterior superior iliac spine, across the inguinal ligament in the subcutaneous plane, and into the femoral incision. If a sufficiently long tunneller is not available, a counter incision may need to be made in the midaxillary line to facilitate tunnelling. It is preferable to avoid such a counter incision to reduce the risk for graft infection. The bypass graft is fixed to the tunnelling instrument and withdrawn from the groin to the subclavicular incision. Polytetrafluoroethylene or Dacron grafts may be used. The diameter selected is based on the diameter of the donor's subclavian artery and usually measures 8 to 10 mm in diameter. Externally ring-supported grafts are preferred because they resist extrinsic compression of the graft against the chest wall and costal margin.

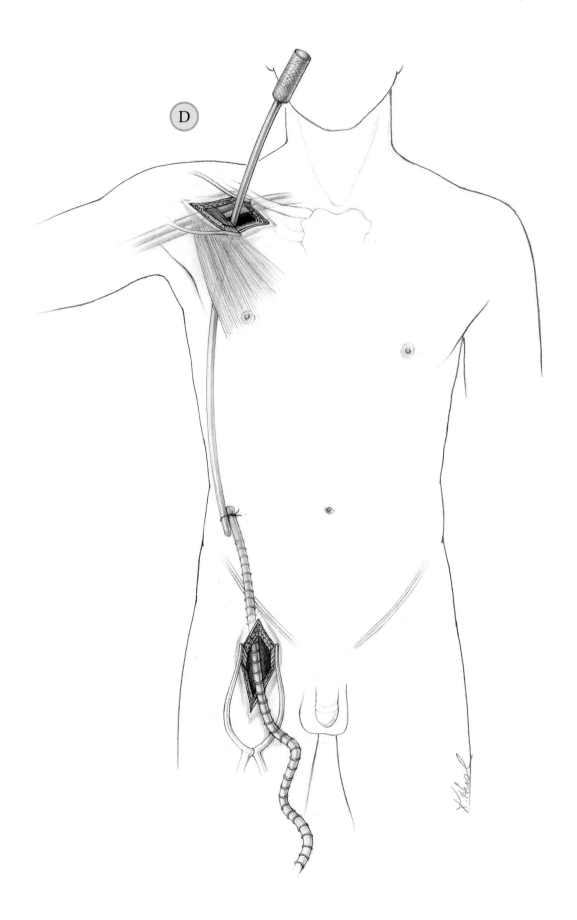

E The proximal anastomosis to the subclavian artery is performed first. Vascular clamps are applied and used to provide a 90-degree torque to the artery. A longitudinal arteriotomy is made just anterior to the highest thoracic artery, which is used as a guide for orientation. The length of the arteriotomy must be precisely the length of the opening in the graft to avoid kinking the subclavian artery when the soft artery is anastomosed to the rigid graft. The anastomosis is performed with 5–0 or 6–0 monofilament nonabsorbable suture and is begun in the middle of the back wall and run in both directions. We prefer to place the graft behind the subclavian vein so that it lies in a more protected place against the chest wall and avoids the possibility of extrinsic compression of the subclavian vein.

F After completion of the anastomosis, a rubbershod clamp is placed on the graft and vascular clamps are released. This allows reperfusion of the right upper extremity and rotation of the artery back to its normal alignment. The graft should then lie posterior to the subclavian vein with no venous compression. Care should be taken to avoid allowing blood to enter the graft before the distal anastomosis is completed so that thrombus does not form along the graft.

G The bypass lies against the chest wall below the pectoralis minor muscle and the subclavian vein.

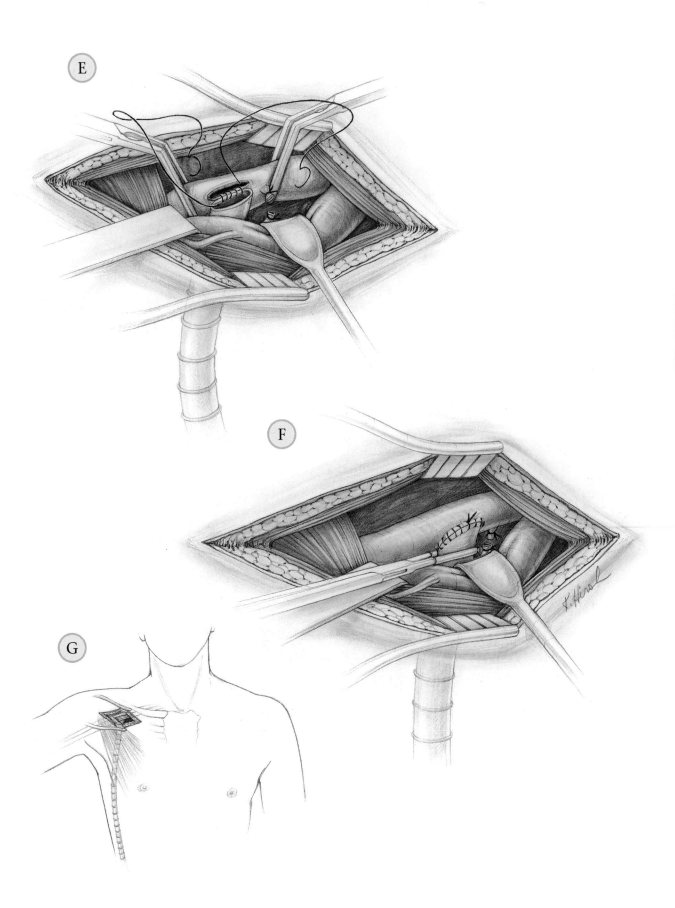

The distal portion of the graft passes anterior to the anterior superior iliac spine and superior to the inguinal ligament to the groin incision.

Vascular clamps are placed on the common femoral, superficial femoral, and profunda femoral vessels, and a longitudinal arteriotomy is made in the common femoral artery. Endarterectomy is performed if necessary, and the arteriotomy may be extended onto the profunda femoris or superficial femoral artery to correct orifice stenoses. The graft is tailored to the arteriotomy and anastomosed using 5–0 monofilament nonabsorbable suture in a running fashion.

After completion of the femoral anastomosis and before allowing blood to enter the graft, a window of graft is removed from the hood of the anastomosis and a ring-supported bypass graft is sutured end-to-side to the distal-most portion of the axillofemoral limb. This anastomosis is performed as distally as possible to maximize the volume flow through the long proximal limb of the bypass graft.

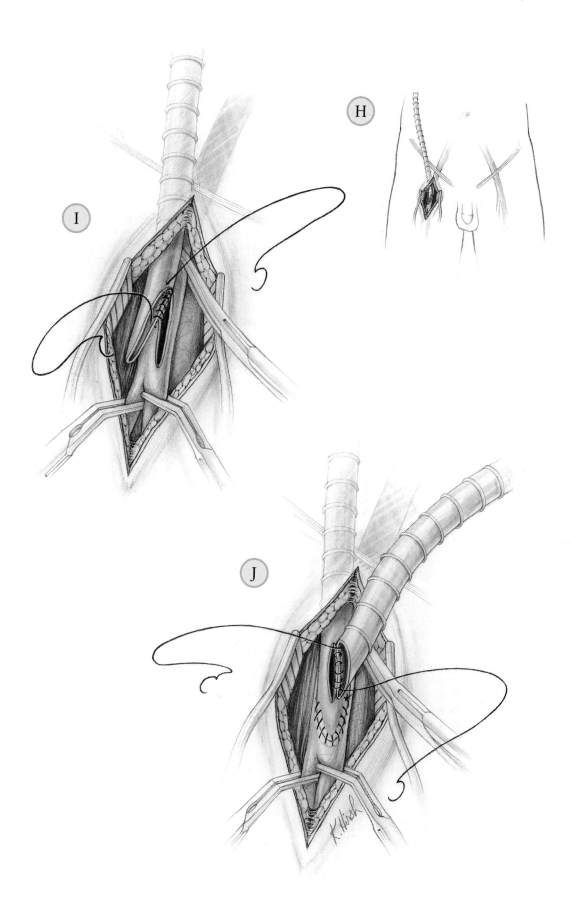

After completion of the anastomoses in the right groin, the proximal clamp on the graft at the subclavian artery is released, and the graft is flushed through the open end of cross femoral limb to evacuate all air from the bypass. The clamp is then replaced, and the distal clamps are removed to allow back bleeding. This maneuver may be done one or more times as necessary to fully flush the system of air and thrombus. A clamp is then placed on the femorofemoral bypass and flow is established to the right leg. The femorofemoral crossover limb is then passed through a suprapubic subcutaneous tunnel to the left groin. This tunnel is created by blunt finger dissection in the subcutaneous plane.

Vascular clamps are then applied to the left femoral artery, and a longitudinal arteriotomy is made in the common femoral artery. Care must be taken in making the arteriotomy and cutting the graft to ensure a good alignment and to avoid kinking of the graft or artery. The femorofemoral bypass is anastomosed to the femoral artery with 5–0 monofilament nonabsorbable suture beginning in the center of the back wall and run in both directions. The bypass is carefully flushed before completion of the anastomosis.

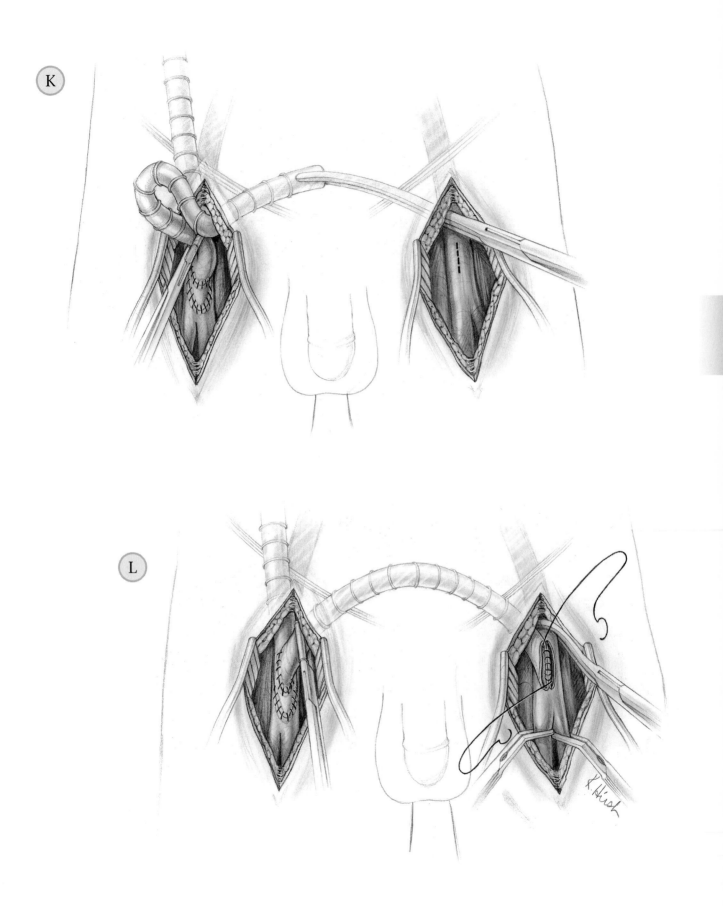

The completed axillofemoral bypass graft is in place. The infected aortic graft has been removed, and the infrarenal aorta and iliac arteries oversewn. Infected grafts may be removed before or after placement of the axillofemoral bypass graft. Removal of the infected aortic graft first has the theoretic advantage of reducing the risk for subsequent infection in the axillofemoral bypass graft. However, this increases the length and complexity of the operation and ensures a period of ischemia after removal of the aortic graft and before completion of the axillofemoral bypass. We usually prefer to place the axillofemoral bypass first and then remove the infected graft either during the same operation or as a secondary staged procedure.

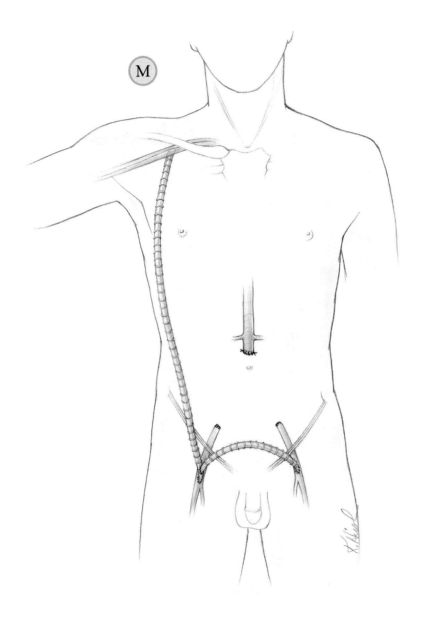

The saphenous vein is the conduit of choice for femoropopliteal bypass grafts. Comparable results are achieved with saphenous vein femoropopliteal bypass grafts when using either the reversed or *in situ* technique.

A

This patient has an occluded right superficial femoral artery and has previously undergone coronary artery bypass graft in which the right saphenous vein was used, and thus is not available for *in situ* bypass. The left saphenous vein is harvested for use as a reversed femoropopliteal bypass. Both legs are prepared and draped from the groin to the ankle. Pads are placed beneath both knees to flex and externally rotate the legs.

B

An incision is made in the right groin for exposure of the common femoral artery. A second incision is made below the right knee for a medial approach to the distal popliteal artery. The tendons of the semimembranosus, semitendinosus, and gracilis muscles are divided. These tendons are not repaired at the completion of the operation and heal without any functional disability to the patient.

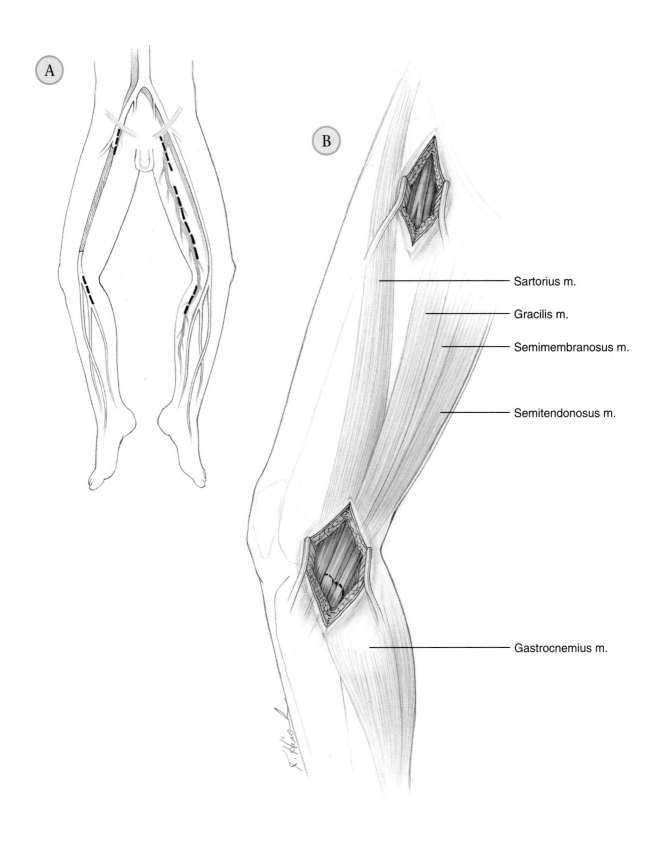

Sartorius m.

Gracilis m.

Semimembranosus m.

Semitendonosus m.

Gastrocnemius m.

The tendon of the medial head of the gastrocnemius muscle is divided and the muscle is retracted posteriorly to expose the distal popliteal artery. This tendon is also not repaired at the end of the procedure.

The popliteal artery lies anterior to the popliteal vein and tibial nerve. A soft portion of the popliteal artery that corresponds to a suitable lumen as demonstrated on preoperative angiography is mobilized and encircled with silastic tapes. Geniculate branches are carefully preserved.

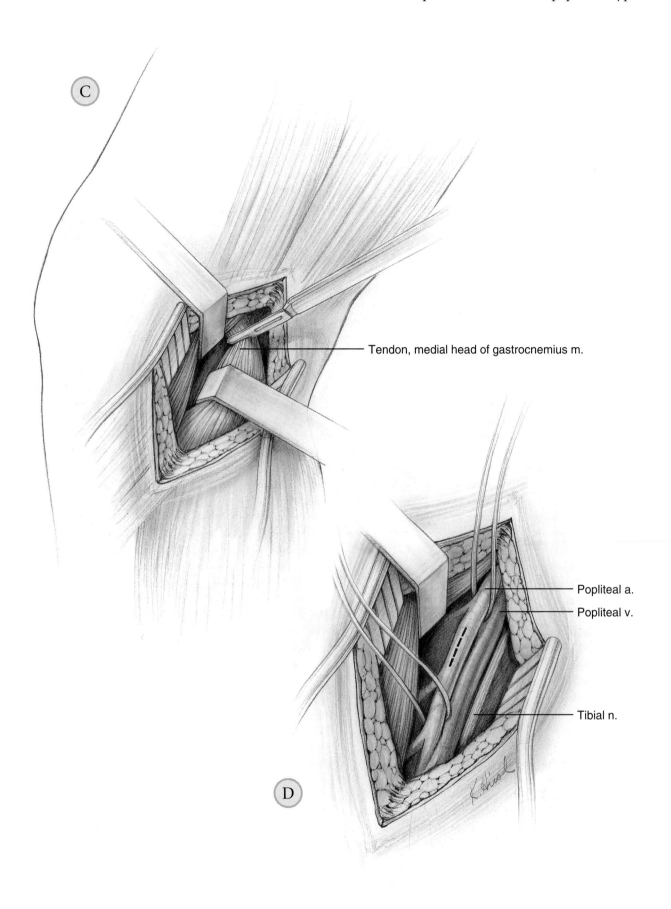

Tendon, medial head of gastrocnemius m.

Popliteal a.

Popliteal v.

Tibial n.

(E) Incisions are made in the left leg directly over the saphenous vein to avoid the creation of skin flaps. The saphenous vein is dissected from the saphenofemoral junction distally until an appropriate length is achieved. To allow better wound alignment, we prefer several interrupted incisions for vein harvest rather than one continuous incision. All side branches are identified, ligated, and divided.

(F) The saphenous vein is excised and flushed with heparinized saline solution to clear blood from the lumen. The lumen is then filled with papaverine and allowed to soak in a papaverine solution to avoid vasospasm. The vein is then flushed to check for leaks. Care is taken to handle the vein gently and to avoid trauma. Only minimal hydrostatic dilation is used.

(G) A tunnelling instrument is passed from the groin beneath the sartorius muscle to the popliteal fossa. The vein is flushed and the tunneller is slowly withdrawn with the vein in a distended position. Passage of the vein in the tunnel in this manner avoids problems of kinking and twisting. The distal portion of the vein is in the groin and the proximal end of the popliteal fossa.

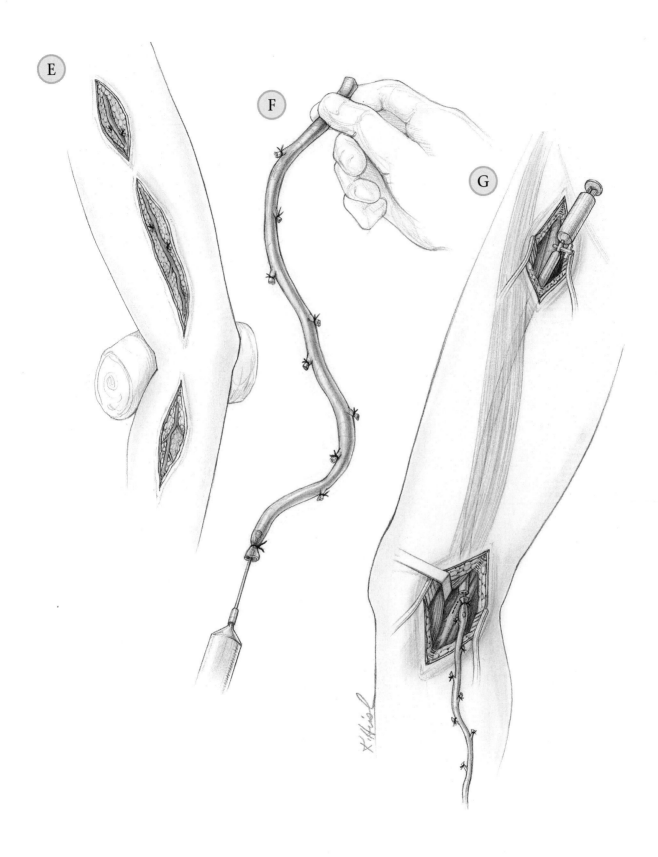

After systemic heparinization, the popliteal artery is clamped. Heifetz clips are most suitable for soft popliteal arteries and minimize the possibility of clamp trauma. However, thick-walled diseased popliteal arteries may require heavier vascular clamps. A longitudinal arteriotomy is made in a soft portion of the popliteal artery. The vein is cut longitudinally for a distance to match the length of the arteriotomy. The anastomosis is begun proximally using 6–0 monofilament suture. A continuous suture technique is used, and each suture is placed under direct vision to ensure that there are no intimal flaps or technical defects.

The corners of the vein are trimmed to avoid creating too large a hood over the anastomosis. The continuous suture line is completed on the side of the anastomosis.

After completion of the distal anastomosis, clamps are placed on the femoral artery, and a longitudinal arteriotomy is made in the common femoral artery. The distal portion of the saphenous vein is spatulated and anastomosed end-to-side to the femoral artery using continuous 6–0 monofilament suture.

The proximal popliteal clamp is removed and flow is established in the saphenous vein bypass. This directs any potential debris into the occluded proximal segment and avoids the possibility of distal embolization. The distal popliteal clamp is then removed and flow is checked using a continuous wave Doppler. A completion arteriogram is obtained to evaluate the distal anastomosis and runoff vessels.

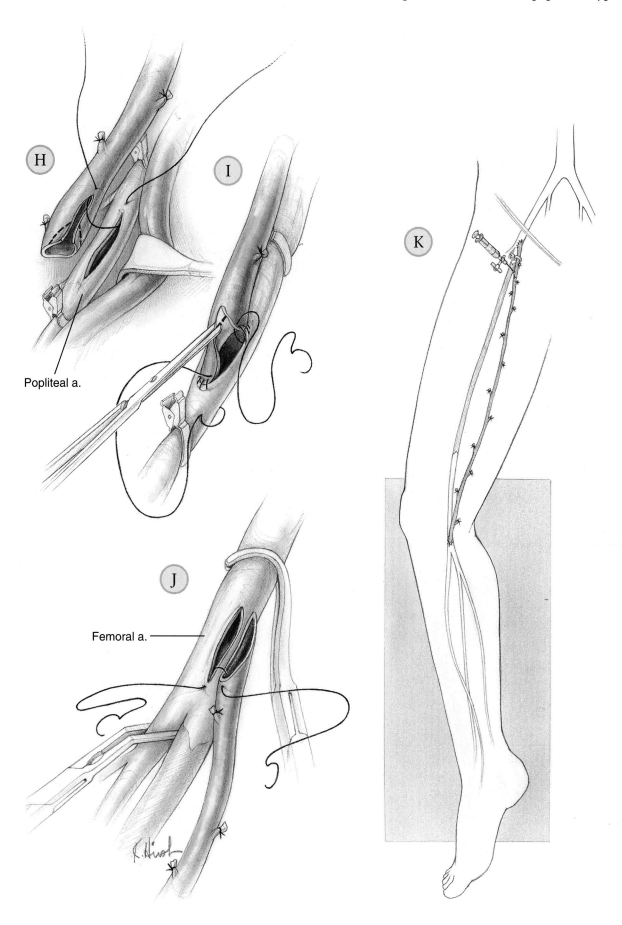

Popliteal a.

Femoral a.

(L) An operative arteriogram demonstrates a tapered contour or "bird's beak" narrowing of a segment of the vein. This may be caused by a torsion or twist, segmental spasm, or other defect. Such defects must be corrected.

(M) Demonstration of a twist of the vein graft that must be repaired.

(N) Twists in the saphenous vein may be corrected by transecting the vein and reanastomosing it end-to-end with a slight spatulation to avoid a focal stenosis.

(O) Operative arteriogram demonstrating a stenosis distal to the anastomosis.

(P) Distal stenoses may be caused by residual plaque distal to the anastomosis or to vascular clamp injury.

(Q) Distal stenoses must be corrected to ensure graft patency. The arteriotomy is extended more distally past the demonstrated lesion and repaired using a vein patch graft.

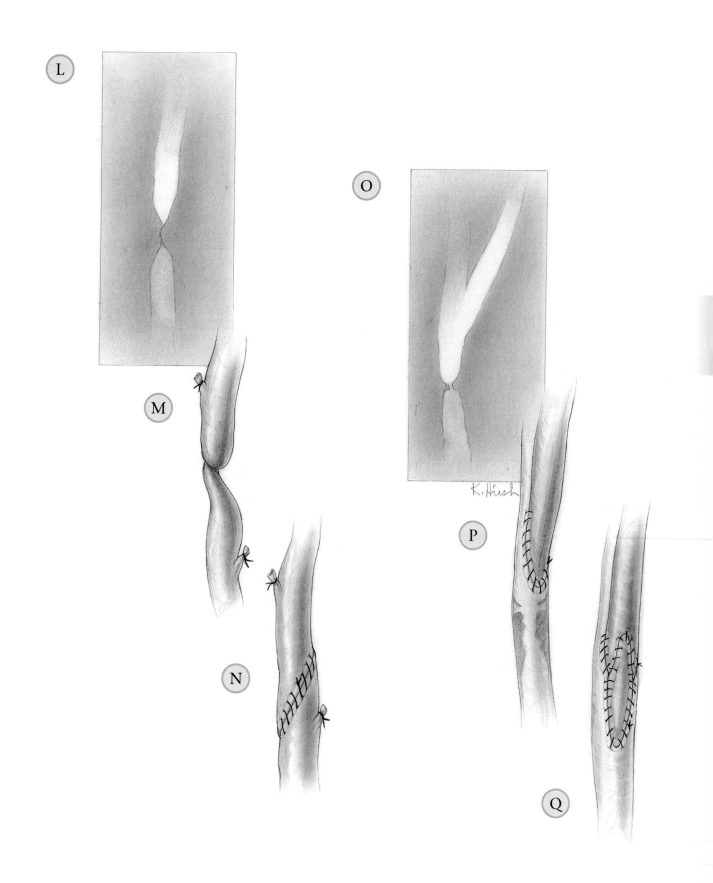

K. Hirsh

Bypasses to the tibial vessels can be performed using a reversed or *in situ* saphenous vein technique. The *in situ* technique has the advantage of suturing the large proximal vein to the common femoral artery and the smaller portion of the distal vein to the distal tibial artery. This is particularly important for distal bypass procedures. The *in situ* technique is attractive because of the size match and because the vein does not need to be removed from its bed. In addition, the *in situ* technique avoids damage to the vein during harvest and torsion or kinking during tunnelling. Finally, the *in situ* technique provides a greater vein utilization rate than the reversed technique because smaller caliber veins can be used.

(A) The patient is placed supine on the operating table, and the leg is prepared from the lower abdomen to the ankle. The leg is externally rotated and supported behind the knee. The patient illustrated has an occluded superficial femoral and proximal popliteal artery. The posterior tibial, anterior tibial, and peroneal arteries are patent. An incision is made in the groin over the saphenofemoral junction, and the proximal saphenous vein is exposed. The entire length of the saphenous vein is exposed on its anterior surface. This can be accomplished through one long incision over the vein or through multiple skin incisions made along the course of the saphenous vein. Multiple incisions heal better but occasionally interfere with visualization of the vein. Visualization and protection of the vein is of utmost importance and one should not hesitate to connect multiple incisions if exposure is impaired.

(B) The proximal saphenous vein is dissected to its junction to the common femoral vein, and branches are ligated and divided. The saphenofemoral junction is fully mobilized and exposed. The adjacent common femoral artery is exposed and control of the common femoral, superficial femoral, and profunda is obtained.

(C) After exposure and control of the posterior tibial artery and distal portion of the saphenous vein, the patient is heparinized. A curved vascular clamp is placed on the femoral vein at the saphenofemoral junction, and the saphenous vein is divided flush with the femoral vein. A Heifetz clip is placed on the saphenous vein for hemostasis. If additional length of vein is needed, a narrow segment of anterior wall of the common femoral vein may be taken with the saphenous vein.

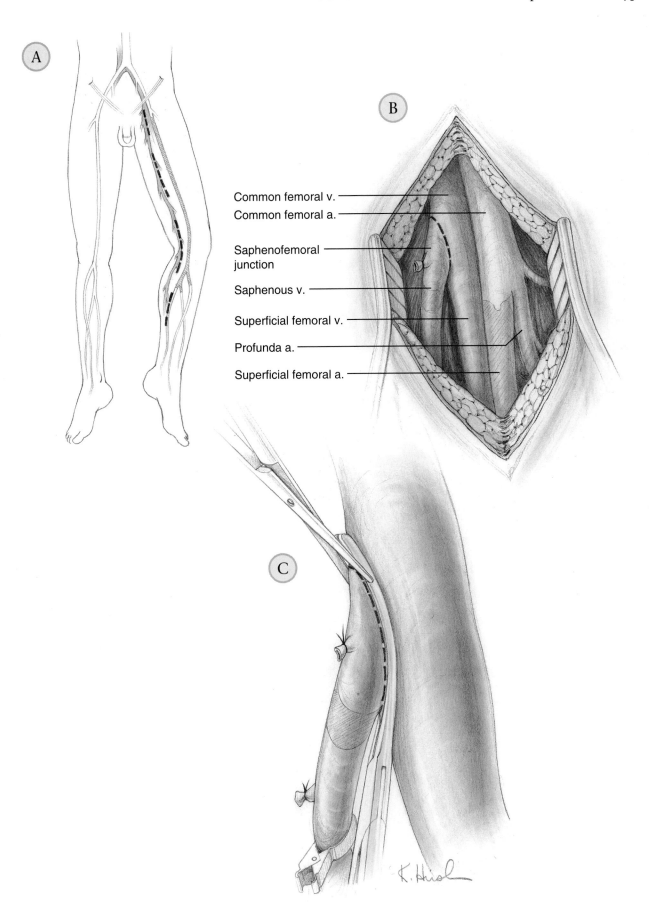

Common femoral v.

Common femoral a.

Saphenofemoral junction

Saphenous v.

Superficial femoral v.

Profunda a.

Superficial femoral a.

The saphenofemoral junction and anterior wall of the femoral vein is closed with continuous 5–0 or 6–0 monofilament suture. The saphenous vein is opened to expose the most proximal valve.

Using loupe magnification and fine scissors, both leaflets of the highest saphenous valve are excised under direct vision.

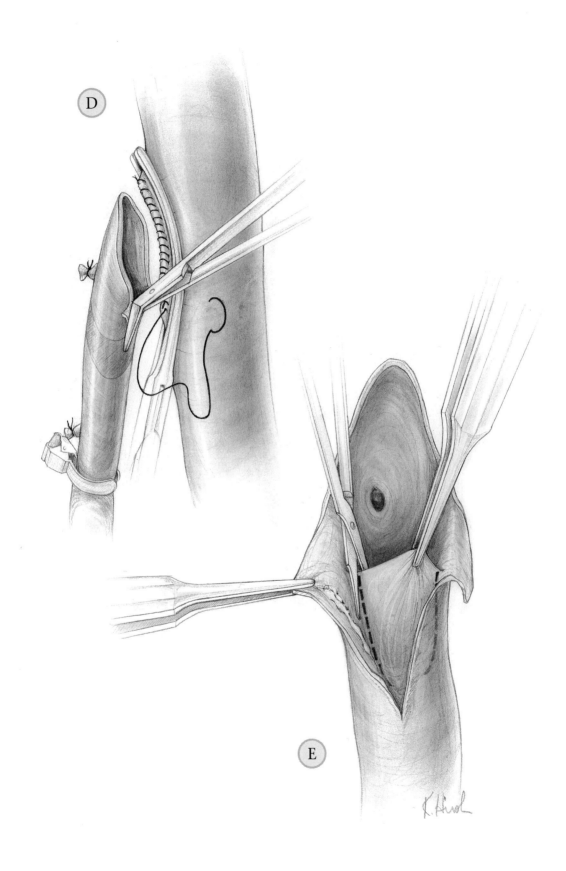

(F) Vascular clamps are applied to the femoral artery, and a longitudinal arteriotomy is made in the common femoral artery. This arteriotomy is made on the anteromedial aspect of the femoral artery to allow proper orientation to the vein that lies medially.

(G) The proximal portion of the vein is anastomosed to the femoral artery using continuous 5–0 or 6–0 monofilament suture.

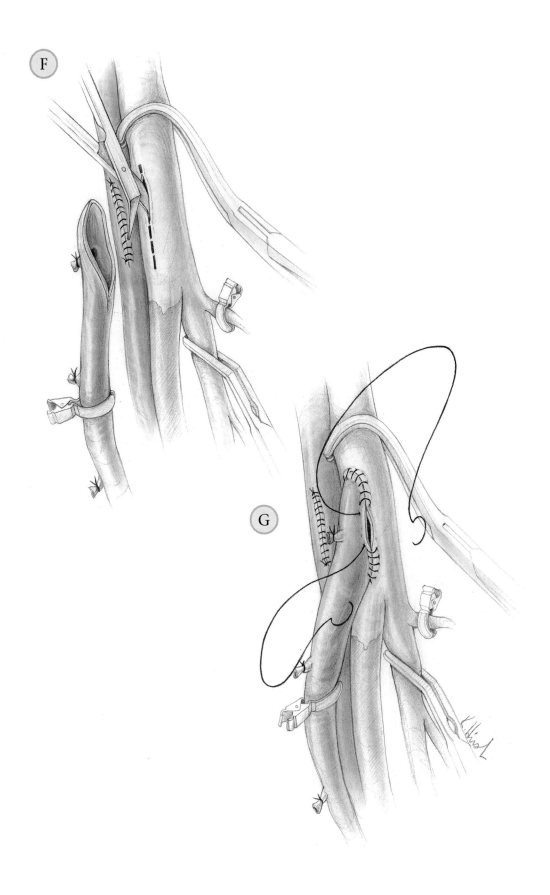

H After completion of the proximal anastomosis, clamps are removed and flow enters the proximal portion of the saphenous vein. Flow stops at the first competent valve; this can usually be identified by the distention of the proximal vein and the collapse of the distal vein. Through large size distal side branches, a valvulotome is introduced and passed proximally through the closed valves. Saphenous vein valves are bicuspid and have anterior and posterior cusps; the plane of closure of the valves is parallel to the skin. Flow of arterial blood through the proximal anastomosis closes the valve cusps; this is essential for valve lysis.

I The valvulotome passes through the cusp in a plane parallel to the skin (parallel to the plane of valve closure) and is then rotated 90 degrees anteriorly.

J The valvulotome is withdrawn, and the tip is carefully observed on the anterior wall of the vein. When a valve is engaged, resistance will be felt. The valvulotome is withdrawn and a sudden release or pop is felt as the cusp is cut.

K The valvulotome is then again advanced in a plane parallel of the skin, past the location of the cut anterior leaflet, rotated 90 degrees posteriorly, and withdrawn to cut the posterior leaflet.

L Both valve cusps are incised and rendered incompetent.

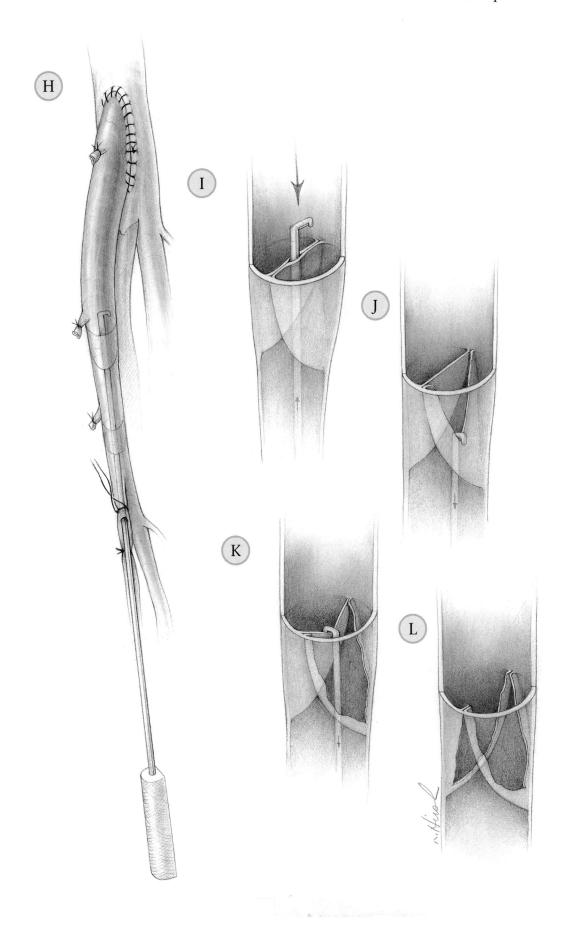

As many side branches are cannulated as necessary to lyse all valves. The final segment of vein is cannulated through the distal cut end of the vein, and successful lysis of all valves is confirmed by a strong pulsatile stream of blood from the end of the vein.

The vein is filled with heparinized saline in a retrograde fashion, and a Heifetz clip is placed on the saphenous vein during anastomosis of the vein to the posterior tibial artery.

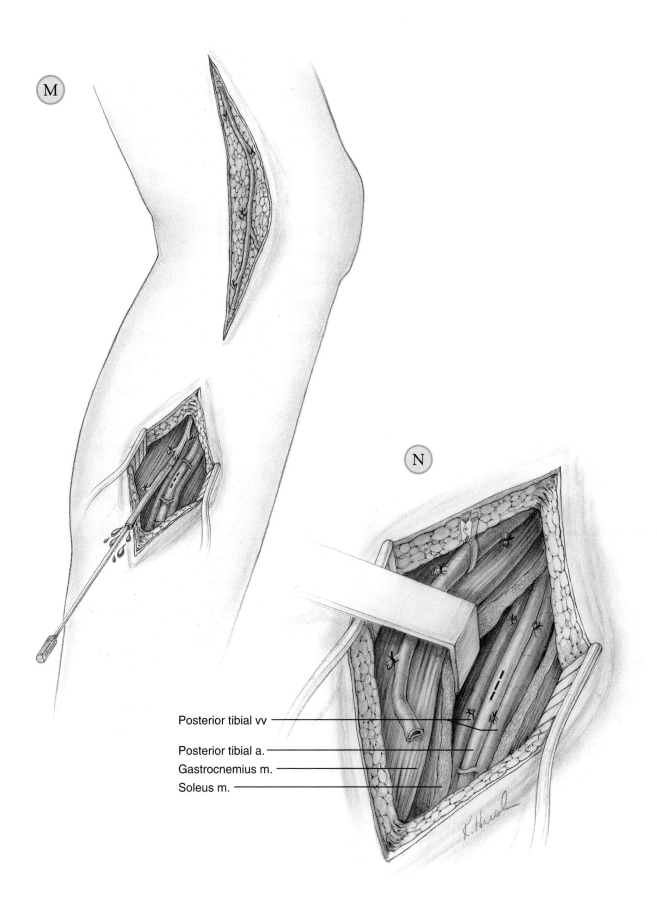

Posterior tibial vv
Posterior tibial a.
Gastrocnemius m.
Soleus m.

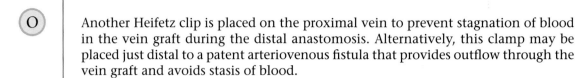

(O) Another Heifetz clip is placed on the proximal vein to prevent stagnation of blood in the vein graft during the distal anastomosis. Alternatively, this clamp may be placed just distal to a patent arteriovenous fistula that provides outflow through the vein graft and avoids stasis of blood.

(P) The distal end of the vein is spatulated and sutured end-to-side to the posterior tibial artery using continuous 6–0 monofilament suture. This anastomosis is performed using magnification with precise visualization of each suture.

(Q) The anastomosis is completed and flow is established to the distal posterior tibial artery. The first outflow is directed retrograde, up the posterior tibial artery to avoid distal embolization of any thrombus material from the inside of the graft.

(R) After flow is established, all remaining side branches and fistulas are ligated. Localization of these fistulas can be facilitated by using an intraoperative Doppler ultrasound. An operative arteriogram is obtained, visualizing the entire length of the graft, as well as the distal anastomosis and outflow tract. Residual arteriovenous fistulas are ligated.

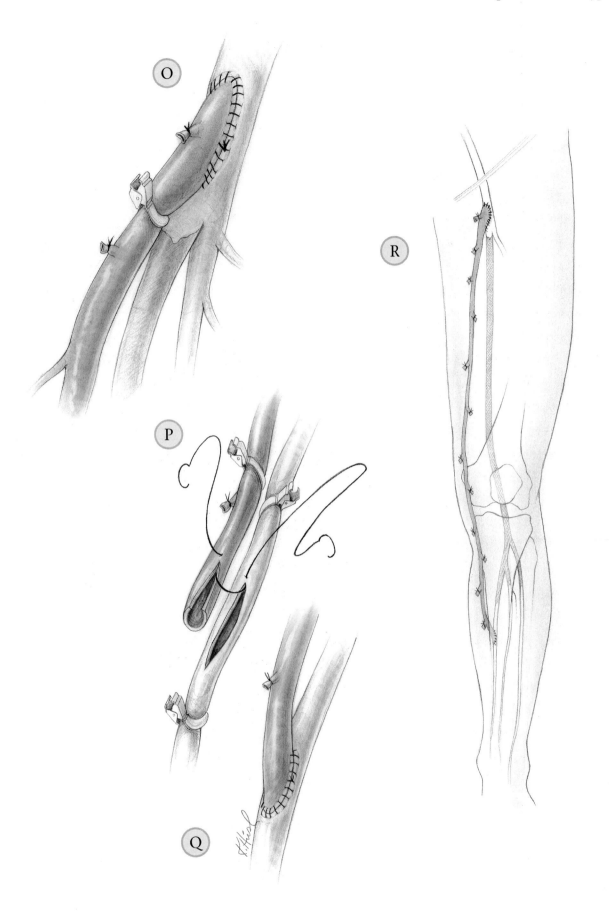

Femoral anterior tibial bypass may be performed using a translocated saphenous vein if the patient has only a short segment of acceptable saphenous vein and a widely patent proximal superficial femoral artery. The vein is not reversed so that the larger proximal portion of the vein can be sutured to the superficial femoral artery, whereas the smaller distal portion of the vein can be sutured to the smaller anterior tibial artery. This requires complete excision of the proximal saphenous vein, translocation of the vein distally, and valve lysis as used in the *in situ* technique.

Incisions are made directly over the saphenous vein from the groin to the knee and laterally in the lower leg over the patent segment of the anterior tibial artery.

The saphenous vein is divided flush with the common femoral vein. The common femoral vein is closed with continuous 5–0 monofilament suture. All side branches of the saphenous vein are divided and ligated, and the saphenous vein is excised from the groin to the knee. The vein is flushed with heparinized saline and placed in a papaverine solution for pharmacologic vasodilation. Through the midthigh incision, the midportion of the superficial femoral artery is mobilized. A soft portion of the artery of satisfactory caliber is chosen for the proximal anastomosis. The anterior tibial artery is exposed at a suitable level as demonstrated by preoperative arteriography.

The highest saphenous valve is excised directly (see page 239), and the proximal end of the vein is anastomosed end-to-side to the superficial femoral artery. Flow is established in the proximal saphenous vein in a retrograde fashion to close the valves. Using a valvulotome, introduced through the end of the vein, all valves are lysed. The vein may be telescoped onto the valvulotome to accommodate its longer length. Pulsatile flow is demonstrated through the end of the saphenous vein. The saphenous vein is placed in its subcutaneous bed medially and tunnelled to the anterior tibial artery laterally either through the interosseous membrane or anteriorly over the tibia in a subcutaneous position. As shown here, the tunnel has been made subcutaneously anterior to the tibia. When the vein is in place in the tunnel and before performing the distal anastomosis, pulsatile flow is again demonstrated through the vein to confirm that no kink has occurred in the tunnel. The distal portion of the vein is then anastomosed end-to-side to the anterior tibial artery in the standard fashion using magnification, 6–0 continuous suture. A completion operative arteriogram is obtained.

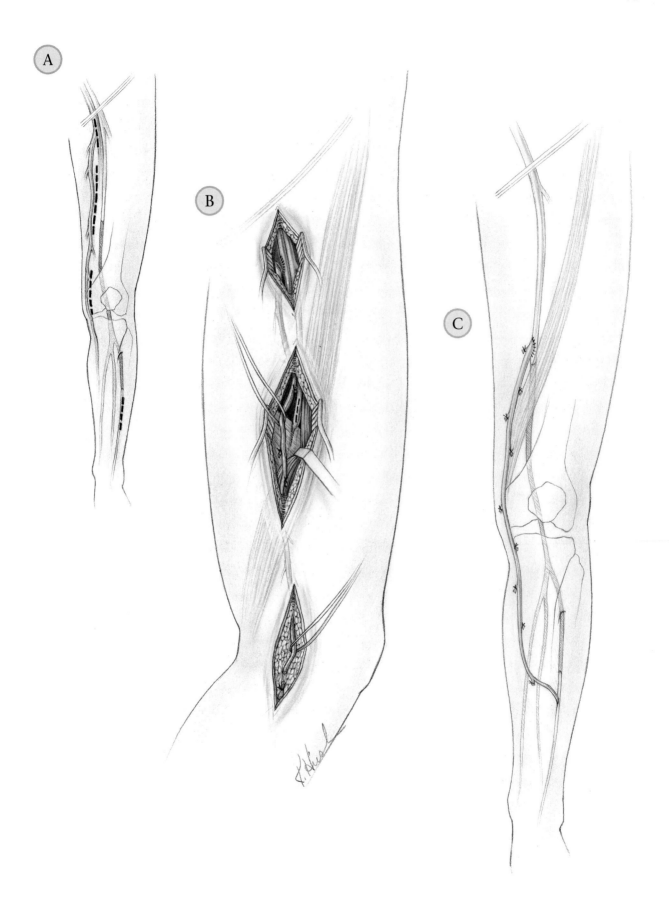

In some circumstances, it may be preferable to tunnel the saphenous vein through the interosseous membrane to the anterior tibial artery. This is particularly true in cases where the vein harvest incision on the medial calf extends to the same level as the lateral incision for exposure of the anterior tibial artery.

A cross section of the midcalf demonstrates the proper tunnel through the interosseous membrane. The anterior tibial artery has been exposed between the tibialis anterior muscle and the extensor digitorum longus muscle. The soleus muscle is detached from the tibia through the medial incision used to harvest the saphenous vein. The interosseous membrane between the fibula and tibia is identified and incised for several centimeters so that a large opening that will not kink the vein graft is produced.

A clamp is passed through the interosseous membrane from medial to lateral. A second clamp can then be passed through the same tract from lateral to medial to grasp the saphenous vein and guide it through the opening.

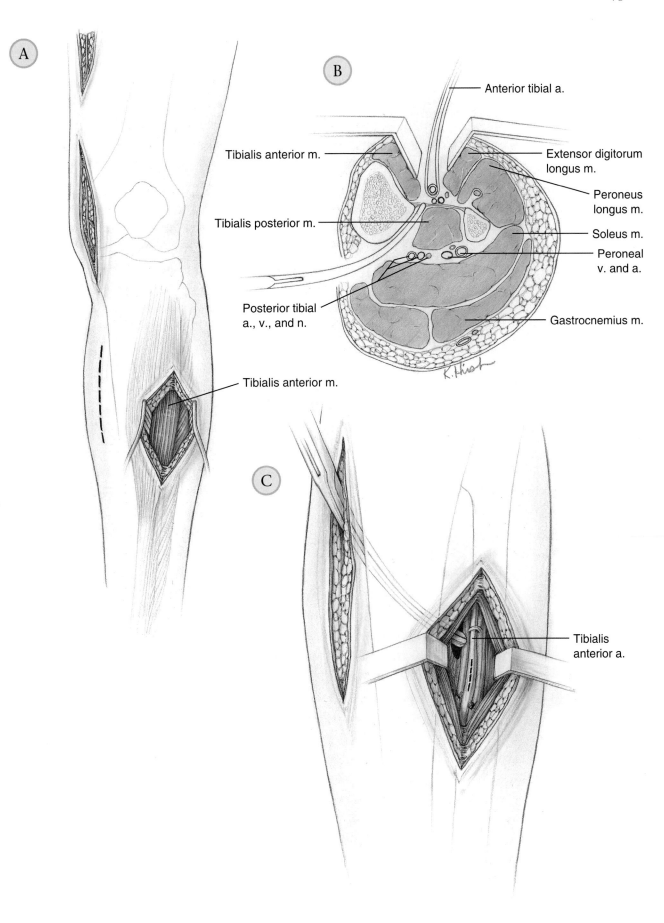

Anterior tibial a.

Tibialis anterior m.

Extensor digitorum longus m.

Peroneus longus m.

Tibialis posterior m.

Soleus m.

Peroneal v. and a.

Posterior tibial a., v., and n.

Gastrocnemius m.

Tibialis anterior m.

Tibialis anterior a.

The saphenous vein is passed through the interosseous membrane. Proximal clamps are removed and blood flow is allowed through the vein to ensure that there are no kinks and to properly adjust the length of the graft. A longitudinal arteriotomy is then made in the anterior tibial artery and the saphenous vein is anastomosed end-to-side to the anterior tibial artery using 6–0 continuous suture and magnification. A completion arteriogram is obtained.

The completed femoral anterior tibial bypass with the vein graft passing through the interosseous membrane to the anterior tibial artery. Passage of the graft through the interosseous membrane is particularly useful when the anastomosis is to be performed to the proximal portion of the anterior tibial artery. Subcutaneous passage of the vein over the anterior portion of the tibia is preferable for anastomoses to the distal portions of the vessel.

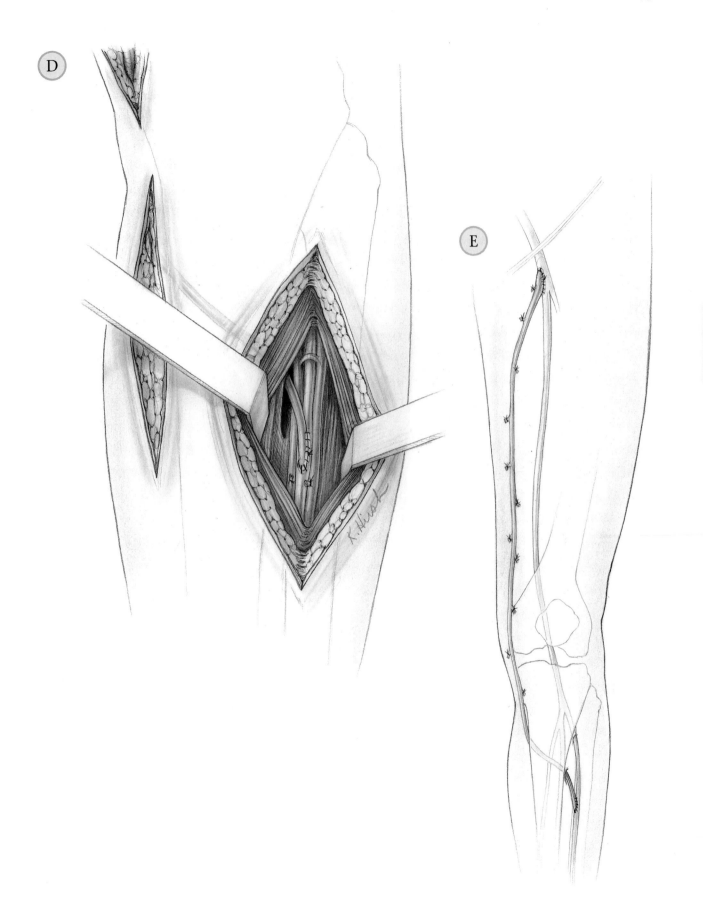

Ⓐ Bypasses to the proximal peroneal artery can be readily accomplished through a medial approach. An incision is made at the medial border of the tibia over the angiographically demonstrated peroneal artery. The soleus muscle is retracted posteriorly and divided at its attachment to the tibia.

Ⓑ The posterior tibial artery and vein are identified. In this instance, the posterior tibial is occluded and not suitable for bypass. Dissection is carried deeper on the underside of the soleus muscle between the soleus and tibialis posterior muscles. The peroneal artery and vein are identified. Suitability of the artery for anastomosis is confirmed by palpation of a soft vessel with a patent lumen. Location of the artery and confirmation of its patency can be facilitated by the use of a Doppler ultrasound probe. If suitability of the vessel is not obvious, intraoperative arteriography should be performed. After identification of a satisfactory outflow vessel, the *in situ* saphenous vein (see pages 239–243) is anastomosed to the peroneal artery in an end-to-side fashion using 6–0 continuous suture and magnification.

Ⓒ The completed femoral peroneal *in situ* saphenous vein bypass. An intraoperative arteriogram is always obtained.

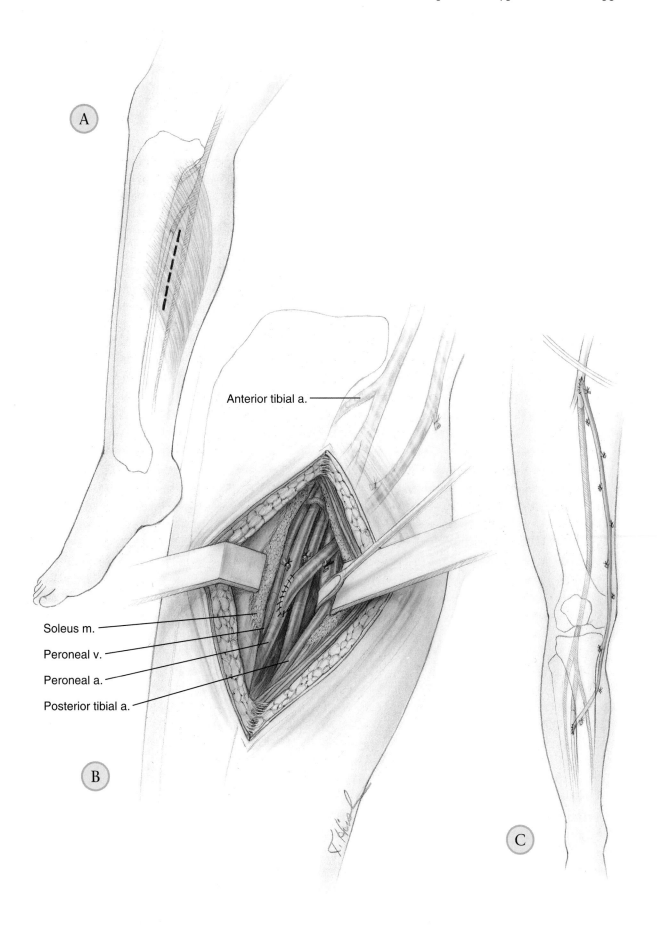

Anterior tibial a.

Soleus m.

Peroneal v.

Peroneal a.

Posterior tibial a.

A

B

C

The distal peroneal artery lies between the tibia and fibula and penetrates the interosseous membrane from posterior to anterior just above the ankle. The distal third of the peroneal artery is difficult to expose through a medial approach and is more readily approached through a lateral approach. Lateral exposure requires a segmental fibulectomy. Removal of the fibula results in no significant functional disability.

(A) Incisions are made over the saphenous vein as previously described for *in situ* bypass (see pages 239–243). An incision is made laterally over the distal third of the fibula.

(B) The periosteum is divided and a periosteal elevator is used to expose the fibula. A Gigli saw is carefully passed around the fibula and a 6-cm segment of fibula is excised. Removal of this portion of the bone results in no impairment of stability or ability to ambulate normally. Care must be taken in removing this portion of the bone because the peroneal artery and veins are located close to the underside of the fibula.

(C) After removal of a segment of fibula, the peroneal artery and vein are identified immediately below the fibula. The saphenous vein is tunnelled from the medial portion of the leg through the interosseous membrane to the peroneal artery where it is anastomosed in an end-to-side fashion using 6–0 continuous suture and loupe magnification.

(D) The completed femorodistal peroneal *in situ* saphenous vein bypass using a lateral approach. An operative arteriogram is obtained to confirm adequacy of the saphenous vein and to evaluate the distal anastomosis and outflow vessels.

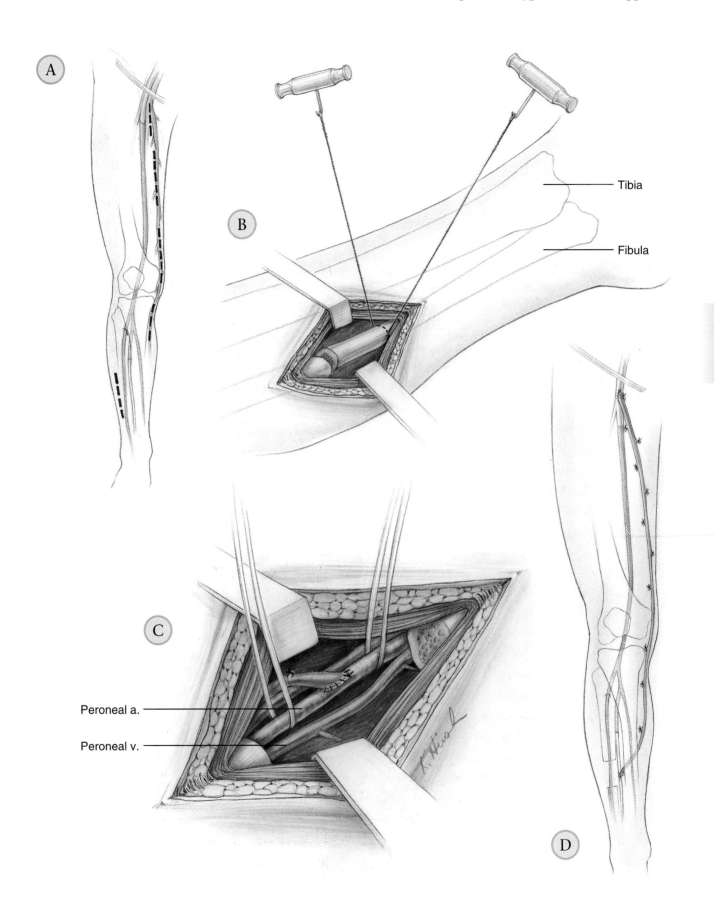

Tibia

Fibula

Peroneal a.

Peroneal v.

Bypasses to the above-knee popliteal artery can be performed using a saphenous vein or prosthetic bypass. If the saphenous vein is not available, we prefer to use a polytetrafluoroethylene prosthetic bypass.

(A) Incisions are made in the groin over the common femoral artery and in the medial thigh over the proximal popliteal artery.

(B) Control is obtained of the common femoral, superficial femoral, and profunda femoral arteries. The sartorius muscle is retracted laterally and the proximal popliteal artery is exposed distal to the adductor hiatus. A blunt tunnelling instrument is passed from the groin to the medial thigh incision beneath the sartorius muscle. The bypass graft is withdrawn through the subsartorial tunnel with care taken to avoid twists or kinks in the graft.

(C) End-to-side anastomoses are made in the common femoral artery and popliteal artery using continuous 5–0 monofilament suture. We prefer to perform the distal anastomosis first followed by the proximal anastomosis. Before completion of the proximal anastomosis, distal clamps are removed to allow back bleeding and to evacuate all air from the graft. Proximal clamps are then released, and the distal anastomosis and outflow vessels are evaluated with a completion arteriogram. Satisfactory function of the graft is confirmed by palpation of the distal pulse and Doppler ultrasound.

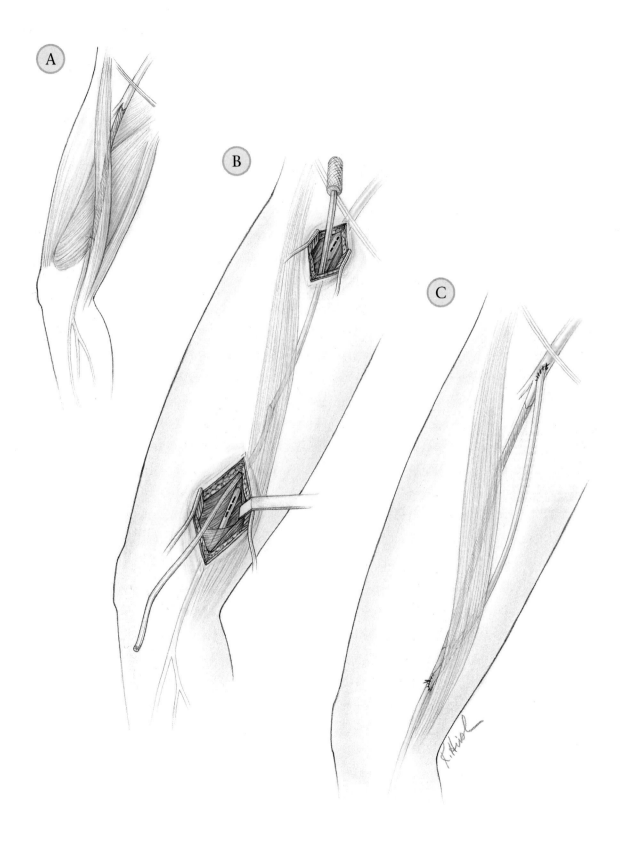

SECTION VI

Reoperative Surgery and Complications

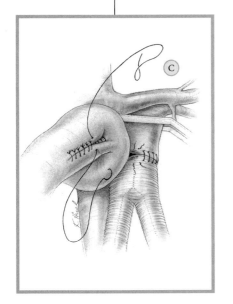

Serious perioperative complications of aortoiliac arterial reconstructions parallel those associated with all major vascular procedures: myocardial events, stroke, renal dysfunction, and pulmonary insufficiency. The incidence of these complications is increased in the high-risk patients undergoing direct aortic reconstructions because of the cardiac stress accompanying intraoperative aortic clamping and postoperative fluid shifts, as well as the expected pulmonary compromise occasioned by abdominal incisions.

Cardiac complications include myocardial infarction, arrhythmias, and congestive heart failure. Prevention of these complications is facilitated by thorough preoperative evaluation and selection of the least stressful procedure (e.g., axillofemoral rather than aortofemoral bypass).

Some degree of renal dysfunction occurs in about 5% to 10% of patients undergoing aortic surgery; the incidence of acute renal failure is considerably lower (1–2%). Preoperative renal insufficiency, reflected in reduced creatinine clearance to less than 40 ml per minute or serum creatinine greater than 2.0 mg per deciliter, is an important risk factor for this complication. The incidence of renal failure can be reduced by ensuring adequate perioperative hydration. Nephrotoxic antibiotics, especially aminoglycosides, should be used sparingly. Many surgeons and anesthesiologists administer an osmotic diuretic such as mannitol (25–50 mg) before aortic clamping. Infusion of low doses of dopamine (2 μg/kg per minute) can also improve renal blood flow and glomerular filtration.

Complications of groin incisions are troublesome immediate problems that can lead to later catastrophe. Hematomas, lymphatic leaks, and even minimal wound separations greatly increase the risk for wound infection and secondary prosthetic graft infection. These complications can be minimized by meticulous hemostasis before careful wound closure in several layers. Although a small volume of lymphatic drainage from the wound in the immediate postoperative period is not uncommon, persistent leakage (for longer than 48 hours) is best treated by wound exploration with ligation of the transected node or duct.

Colonic ischemia is more common after aortic aneurysmectomy but can occur after aortic reconstruction for occlusive disease, especially in the presence of extensive mesenteric and internal iliac artery disease. As noted earlier, every attempt should be made to maintain internal iliac and inferior mesenteric artery flow. This may require end-to-side rather than end-to-end proximal anastomoses in selected cases and avoidance of any injury to the inferior mesenteric artery.

Ischemia most commonly involves the left colon and classically presents 24 to 72 hours after surgery. Patients experience diarrhea with microscopic or gross blood. It is critical that the diagnosis is established immediately by sigmoidoscopy at the bedside. Laparotomy is indicated if mucosal ischemia is severe, consistent with transmural injury. Treatment of lesser degrees of ischemia includes antibiotics, discontinuation of vasopressors, maximization of cardiac output with fluids, and the use of minimal pain medication to increase the validity of frequent physical examinations. Surgery should be performed if diarrhea, leukocytosis, and pain persist, or if obvious signs of peritonitis or perforation appear.

Aortoduodenal fistulae may develop as a late complication of aortic reconstruction by erosion of a proximal anastomotic pseudoaneurysm into the duodenum or breakdown of the duodenum caused by contact with the proximal suture line. The leakage of duodenal contents leads to secondary infection of the graft and eventual disruption of the anastomosis. In rare instances, the graft may be uninfected, and closure of the duodenum and segmental aortic graft replacement may be possible. Usually, this is not the case, and the graft must be removed and extraanatomic bypass is performed.

Patients with aortoduodenal fistula characteristically present with recurrent, self-limited episodes of upper gastrointestinal hemorrhage, thus providing time to perform diagnostic studies. If untreated, massive gastrointestinal hemorrhage eventually occurs and mandates emergency surgery. Any patient who has previously undergone aortic grafting and experiences gastrointestinal bleeding, with or without back pain or low-grade fever, should be urgently evaluated with aortography, computed tomography scanning, and upper gastrointestinal endoscopy.

(A) The duodenum is usually adherent to the proximal aortic anastomosis with a variable degree of inflammation. If significant inflammation or pseudoaneurysm formation is present, the supraceliac aorta is controlled at the aortic hiatus (see pages 85 and 119) before mobilizing the duodenum.

(B) The patient is systemically heparinized and the infrarenal aorta is encircled proximal to the aortic anastomosis. If there is insufficient length of infrarenal aorta, suprarenal aortic control is obtained. The duodenum is separated from the aortic anastomosis; leakage of duodenal contents is minimized by pinching the fistula closed. The edges of the duodenal defect are debrided.

(C) The duodenum is repaired in two layers using a running inner layer of absorbable suture and an interrupted, inverting outer layer of 3–0 nonabsorbable suture. In this case, the aortic graft is seen to be bile stained and is poorly incorporated confirming the presence of graft infection and the need for graft excision.

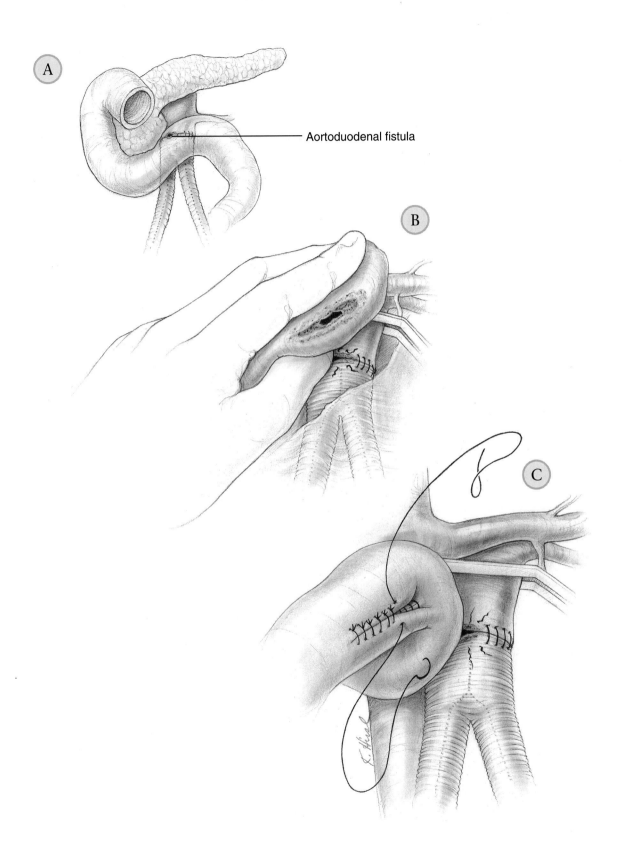

Aortoduodenal fistula

D   The proximal aorta is debrided to the level of normal aorta. Failure to completely debride friable and infected aortic wall will result in continuing infection and blowout of the aortic stump. If necessary, the infrarenal clamp should be moved to a suprarenal position to facilitate debridement of the aorta to the level of the renal arteries.

E   The aortic stump is closed with two layers of continuous 3–0 monofilament suture. Large, deep bites should be taken to obtain a secure closure.

F   Occasionally, a flap of prevertebral fascia may be used to buttress closure of the aortic stump. Mattress sutures are placed using the fascial patch as a pledget. This maneuver is helpful in achieving a secure closure, but it does not replace adequate debridement of infected aortic tissue.

   The remainder of the infected graft is removed, and suction drains are left in place in the retroperitoneal space.

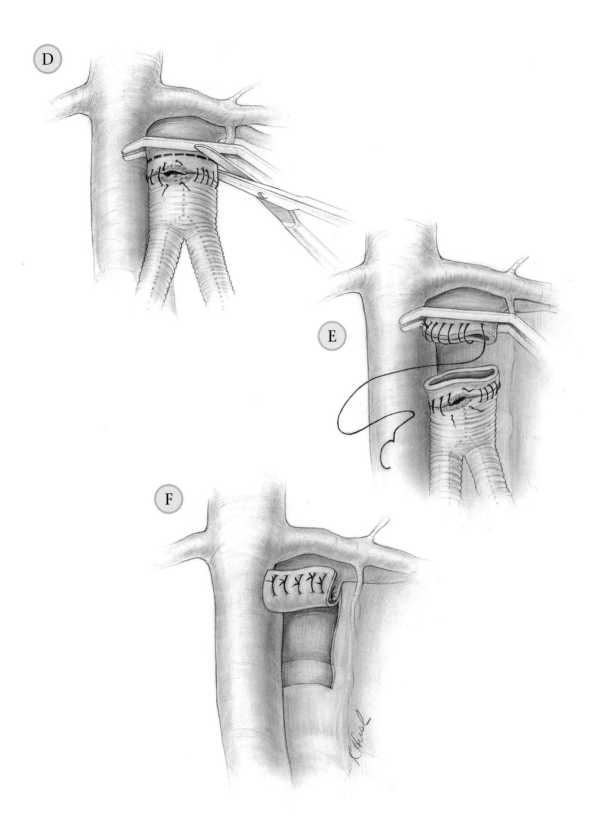

Patients may have localized infections involving only one limb of an aortofemoral bypass. Most commonly this is a sequela of a postoperative wound infection after the aortofemoral bypass that involved only one groin. Patients with a groin mass consistent with a pseudoaneurysm, inflammatory mass, or draining sinus after aortofemoral bypass should be studied with computed tomography scanning and arteriography. These studies will detect pseudoaneurysms at other anastomoses, evaluate distal vessels, and ascertain whether there is fluid collected around the aortic portion of the graft. If these studies reveal no evidence of infection in the body of the graft, plans may be made for local excision of the infected segment.

The patient is positioned on the operating table for a left flank incision; the draining left groin is draped out of the operative field. The left limb of the graft is exposed through a left flank retroperitoneal approach.

The left limb of the graft is identified and exposed. Particular care is taken to avoid injury to the left ureter that crosses over the graft. The proximal-most portion of the left limb of the graft is carefully inspected for signs of graft infection. If there is poor incorporation of the graft or if the graft is surrounded by purulent material that tracks up to the body of the aortic graft, it must be assumed that the entire graft is infected. Under these circumstances, the entire graft must be removed. If, however, the graft is well incorporated and not surrounded by fluid, the graft is transected close to its origin and oversewn proximally with continuous monofilament suture. A segment of graft from this area is excised and sent for aerobic and anaerobic bacterial culture. The distal end of the graft is oversewn with monofilament vascular suture. The abdominal wound is closed and sterile dressings are applied.

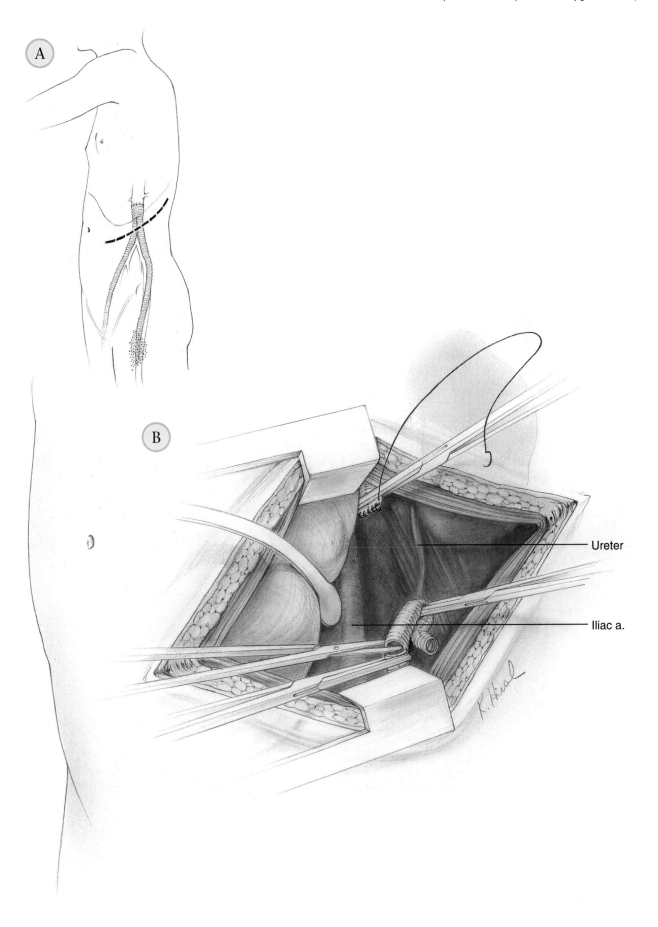

Ureter

Iliac a.

(C) The flank incision is draped out of the operative field, and the left groin is exposed. The previous groin incision is reopened, and the left limb of the graft, common femoral, superficial femoral, and profunda vessels are dissected. The left limb of the graft is withdrawn into the wound through the retroperitoneal tunnel.

(D) The femoral artery is clamped, and the anastomosis of the graft to the femoral artery is excised. A rim of femoral artery is removed with the anastomosis, and any infected femoral artery wall is debrided.

(E) The common femoral artery is closed with a saphenous vein patch. If the femoral artery is disrupted or if groin inflammation and purulence is extensive, total incision of the infected femoral artery with suture ligation of the common femoral, superficial femoral, and profunda femoral arteries is necessary.

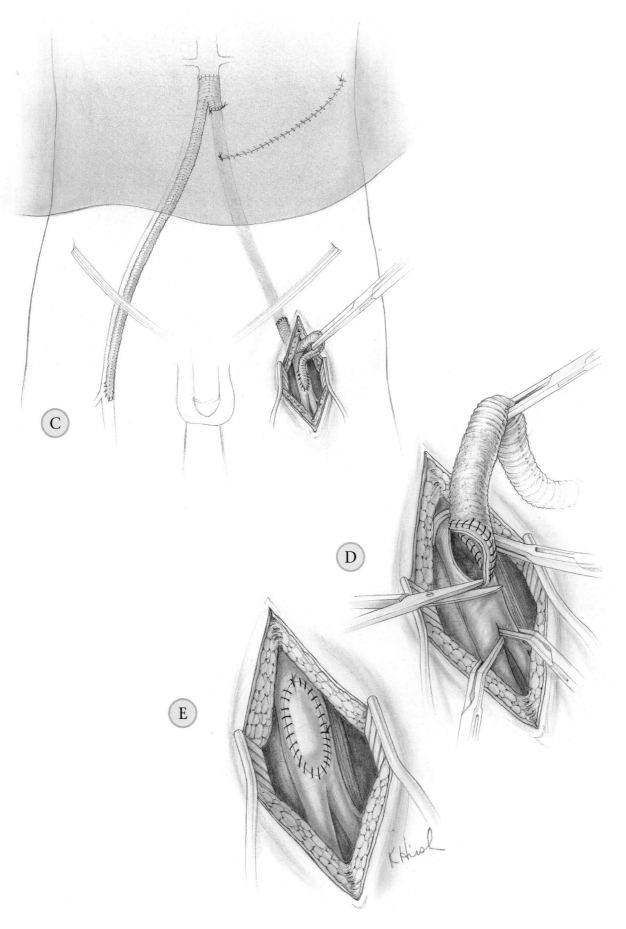

A closed suction drainage catheter is left in the retroperitoneal tunnel. The groin wound is debrided. The femoral artery may be covered by mobilizing the sartorius muscle mediallv. The sartorius muscle should not be used to cover inadequately debrided tissue; this would result in a closed space infection.

If the viability of the left leg is in question, revascularization should be performed. The left groin wound is dressed and excluded from the surgical area. After appropriate preparation and draping, incisions are made in the right groin and left thigh over an acceptable outflow vessel as demonstrated by preoperative arteriography. The incision should be a distance from the infected wound. Anastomoses may be performed to either the profunda or superficial femoral arteries in their mid or distal portions. A right to left femorofemoral bypass is then performed. The proximal anastomosis of the femorofemoral bypass is to the right limb of the aortofemoral bypass in the right groin. We prefer externally supported polytetrafluoroethylene or Dacron grafts. The graft is tunneled subcutaneously to the left leg avoiding the infected groin wound.

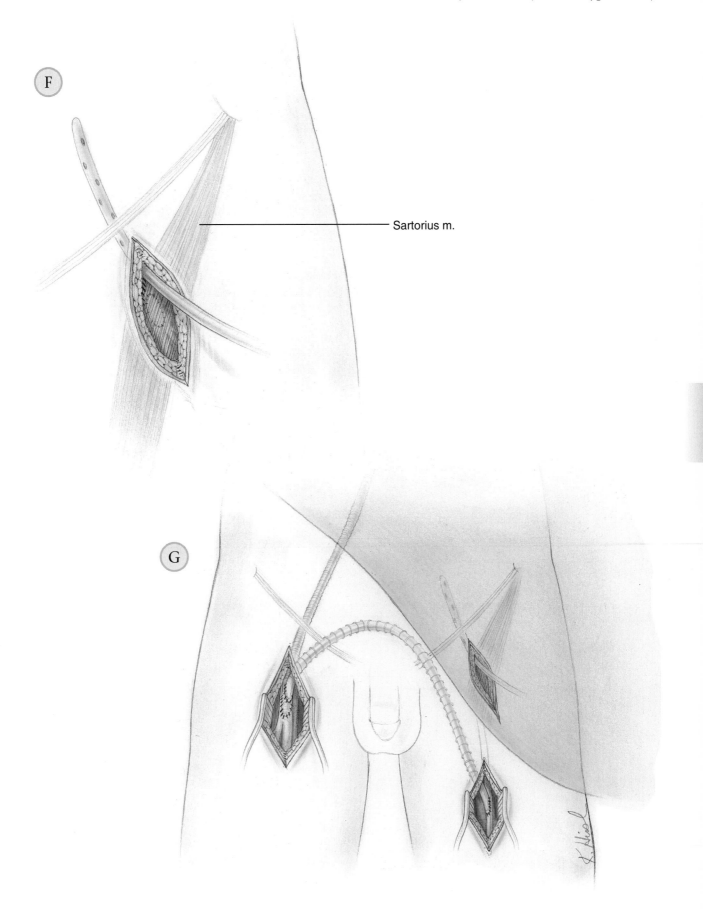

Sartorius m.

Anastomotic pseudoaneurysms of the femoral artery after aortofemoral bypass may be caused by disruption of the suture line, excess tension at the anastomosis, artery wall degeneration, and infection. Pseudoaneurysms that are not infected are repaired by interposing a new segment of prosthetic graft between the aortofemoral bypass limb and patent distal arteries. Preoperative arteriography is useful to identify out-flow vessel patency.

(A)

Most femoral pseudoaneurysms can be repaired through the previous groin inci-sion. In cases where the pseudoaneurysm is large and extends above the inguinal ligament, a suprainguinal incision for retroperitoneal control of the aortofemoral by-pass may be necessary.

(B)

The pseudoaneurysm is exposed anteriorly, and control is obtained of the right limb of the aortofemoral bypass above the aneurysm. After systemic heparinization, the graft is cross-clamped and the aneurysm is opened. If there is significant scarring in the groin or the aneurysm is entered before the aortofemoral bypass is controlled, digital pressure is applied at the inguinal ligament and the bypass graft is identifed and clamped within the pseudoaneurysm. No effort is made to dissect the superfi-cial femoral or profunda branches. They are both easily controlled from within the aneurysm with balloon catheters. The right limb of the aortofemoral bypass is tran-sected, the distal anastomosis is excised, and the distal graft segment is removed. A segment of the graft is sent for aerobic and anaerobic cultures.

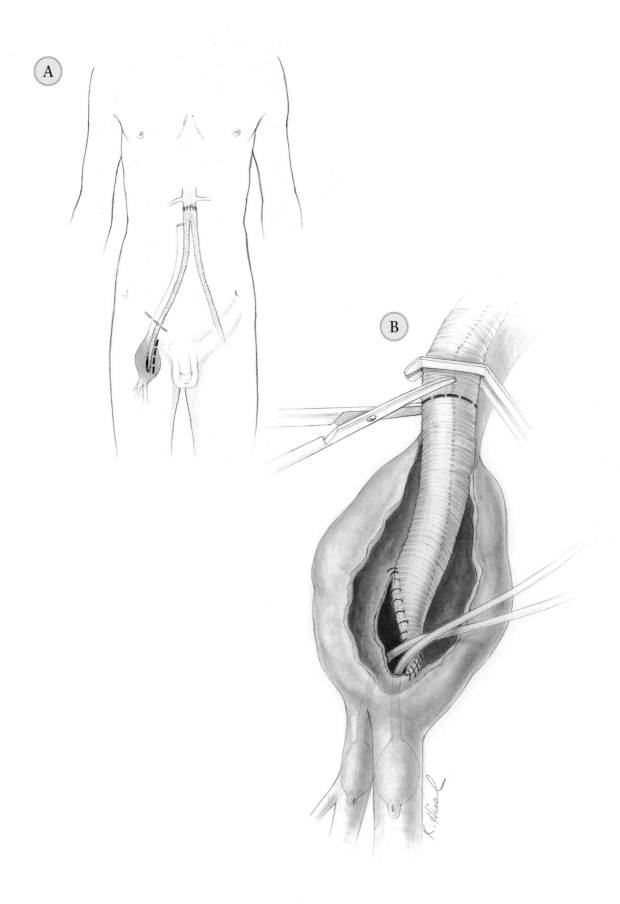

The orifice of the native common femoral artery is oversewn from within the aneurysm.

A new segment of Dacron graft, of appropriate diameter to match to original graft limb, is sutured to the orifice of the superficial femoral and profunda arteries. Large, deep bites are taken to ensure a full-thickness passage of each suture. At times it is helpful to transect the back wall of the common femoral artery to facilitate placement of the posterior wall sutures.

After completion of the distal anastomosis, the balloon catheters are removed and a clamp is placed on the Dacron graft for hemostasis. The new graft is then anastomosed end-to-end to the original Dacron graft using a continuous monofilament suture.

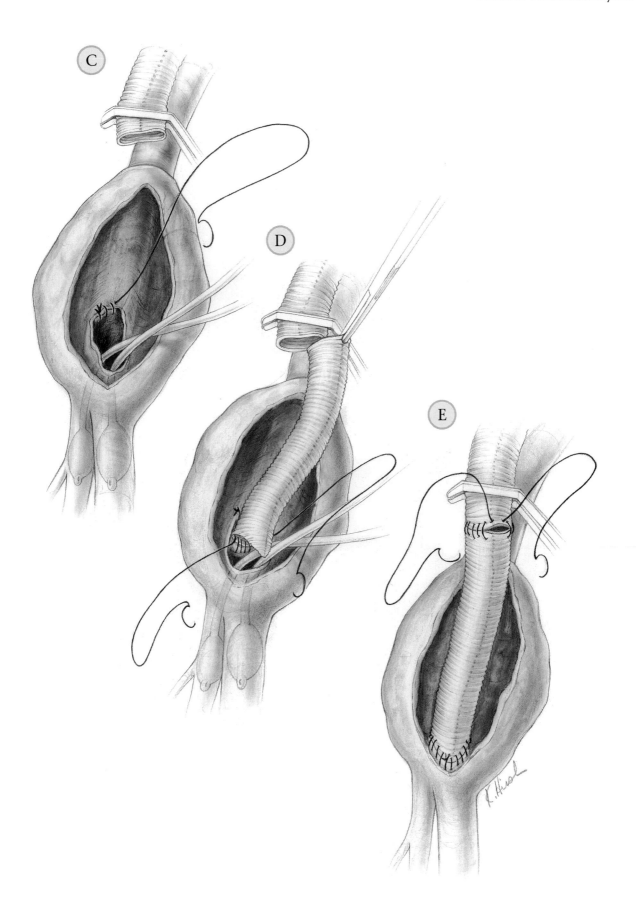

Thrombectomy of acutely occluded saphenous vein bypasses may be successful in restoring patency if performed early.

(A) The proximal and distal anastomoses are exposed through the previous incisions. The patient is systemically heparinized, and the femoral artery is clamped. Longitudinal incisions are made in the saphenous vein over the hood of the anastomosis.

(B) The proximal anastomosis is inspected, and thrombus is removed. A balloon thromboembolectomy catheter is passed down the length of the vein, and thrombus is extracted.

(C) The balloon catheter is then passed proximally and distally in the distal artery to establish brisk back bleeding.

(D) The cause of vein graft occlusion must then be determined. Intraoperative angiography of the thrombectomized vein is performed to detect sclerotic valves, stenoses, or residual thrombus material. A frequent problem is stenosis of the most distal portion of *in situ* vein bypasses. This can be visualized by extending the longitudinal incision in the vein graft past the area of stenosis.

(E) The stenosis is corrected using a saphenous vein patch sewn in with continuous vascular suture.

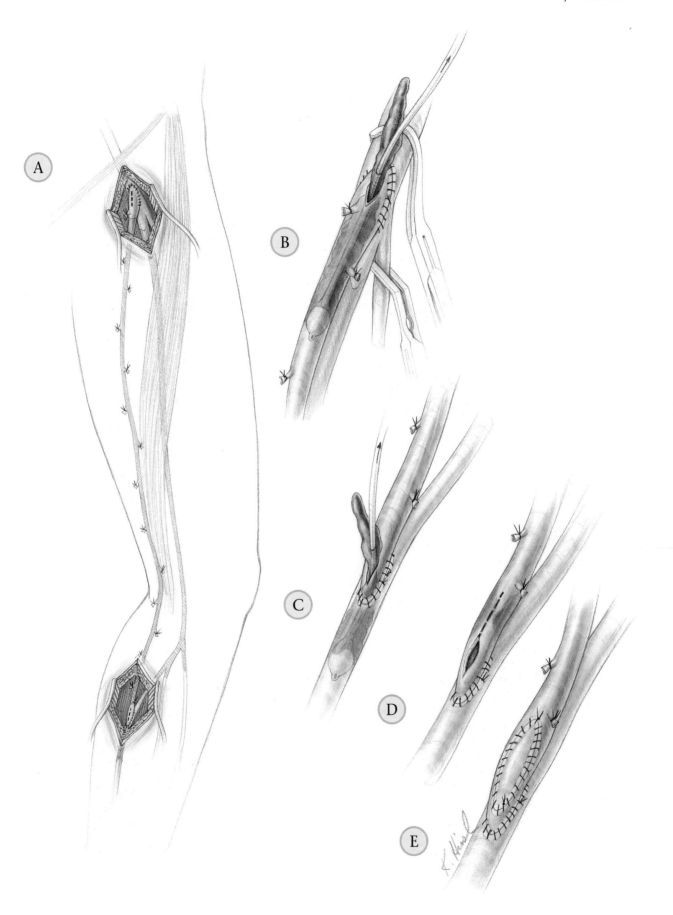

Anastomotic intimal hyperplasia frequently occurs at the distal anastomosis of by-pass grafts. Developing stenoses can sometimes be detected before graft occlusion by serial ankle–brachial pressure index measurements and Duplex imaging of the graft and distal anastomosis. Angiography will fully define the graft status. Correction of stenoses before graft occlusion occurs can prevent graft thrombosis.

(A) The distal anastomosis is exposed, and control is obtained of the graft. The artery is exposed for a distance past the anastomosis to a normal, soft segment. The hood of the graft is opened, and the anastomosis is inspected.

(B) The arteriotomy is extended past the area of intimal hyperplasia, and the hyperplastic lesion is removed using a spatula.

(C) A new monofilament suture is placed on either side of the arteriotomy. The original suture is tied to the new suture to prevent unraveling of the original suture line.

(D) A vein patch is used to close the arteriotomy.

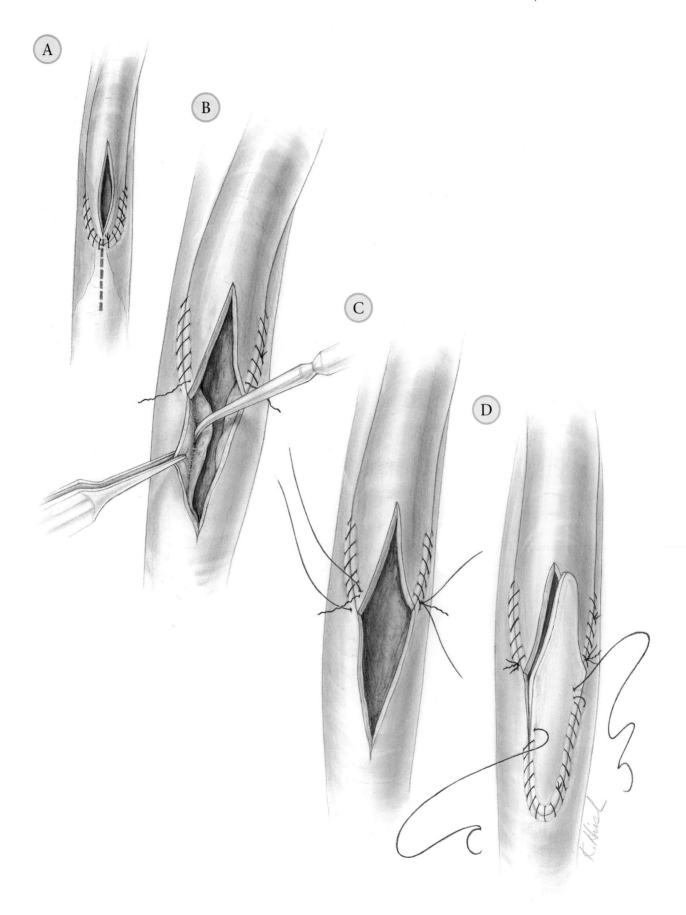

Occasionally, diffuse fibrosis and intimal thickening of a saphenous vein bypass will lead to its occlusion without anastomotic intimal hyperplasia. Under these circumstances, the bypass can be replaced with a prosthetic bypass graft while still using the satisfactory distal anastomosis.

(A) After obtaining control of the distal artery and occluded vein bypass, the saphenous vein graft is amputated. The vein is opened on its anterior aspect to fully expose the anastomosis.

(B) The anastomosis is inspected to confirm the absence of intimal hyperplasia. The prosthetic graft is anastomosed end-to-end to the previous vein bypass using continuous monofilament suture.

(C) The artery is allowed to back bleed, and the graft is flushed to evacuate all air and debris before completion of the anastomosis. A completion arteriogram is obtained.

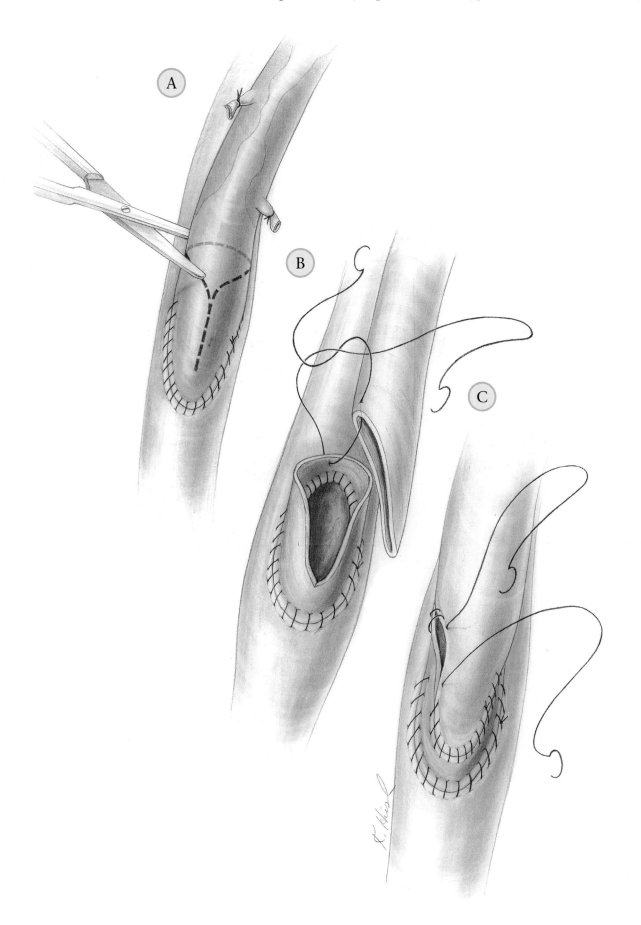

Index

Page numbers followed by f represent figures.

Semitendinosus muscle, 226, 227f
Sigmoid colon, 72
Soleus muscle
in femoral anterior tibial bypass, 245f, 251f
in femoroperoneal bypass, 254, 255f
Spinal cord blood flow, 123
Splenic artery, 187f
Splenorenal bypass, 158, 162, 163f
Stents
in abdominal aortic aneurysm repair, 88, 89, 96, 97f, 98, 99f, 100, 101f, 102, 103f, 104, 105f
balloon dilation in, 106, 107f
for thoracic aortic aneurysm repair, 123
Sternocleidomastoid muscle
in carotid endarterectomy, 6, 7f
small artery to, 7f
in subclavian artery revascularization, 40, 41f
in subclavian to external carotid bypass, 32, 33f
in vertebral artery revascularization, 46, 47f
Stroke, 4
Styloid process, 6
Subclavian artery
in axillofemoral bypass, 214, 215f
to carotid bypass, 32, 33f, 40, 44, 45f
in innominate endarterectomy, 52, 53f
revascularization of, 40, 41f, 42, 43f
in thoracoabdominal aortic aneurysm repair, 125f
in vertebral artery revascularization, 46, 47f, 48, 49f
Subclavian vein, 214, 215f
Superficial femoral artery
in aortofemoral bypass, 196, 197f
in femoral aneurysm repair, 136, 137f
in femoral posterior tibial bypass, 236, 237f
in popliteal aneurysm repair, 140, 141f
Superficial femoral vein, 237f

Superior laryngeal nerve
in carotid endarterectomy, 6, 7f
injury to, 5
Superior mesenteric artery (SMA)
embolectomy, 174, 175f, 176, 177f
endarterectomy, 190, 191f
in mesenteric bypass procedure, 179f
in thoracoabdominal aortic aneurysm repair, 127f
in transaortic visceral artery endarterectomy, 187f
Superior mesenteric bypass, 178, 179f, 180, 181f, 182, 183f
Superior mesenteric vein (SMV), 175f, 179f
Superior thyroid artery
in carotid endarterectomy, 6, 7f, 8, 9f
in internal carotid angioplasty, 30, 31f
Suprarenal aortic aneurysms, 84, 85f
Suturing. See also specific procedures.
in aortofemoral bypass, 200, 201f
in carotid endarterectomy, 10, 11f, 12, 13f
Sympathetic ganglion, 46, 47f

T

Testicular vein, 148, 149f
Thoracic artery, 214, 215f
Thoracic duct, 40
Thoracoabdominal aortic aneurysms, 122-133
anatomical exposure for, 123, 124, 125f, 126, 127f
atriofemoral bypass in, 132, 133f
balloon catheterization in, 126
classification of, 122, 123
closure of, 130, 131f
endoluminal devices for, 123
grafting and anastomoses in, 128, 129f, 130, 131f, 132, 133f
principles in repair of, 123
risk for rupturing, 122
Thrombosis
superior mesenteric artery, 171, 172
vein graft, 278, 279f

Thyrocervical trunk
in subclavian artery revascularization, 41f, 42, 43f
in vertebral artery revascularization, 46, 47f
Tibia, 256, 257f
Tibial artery
anterior
in femoral anterior tibial bypass, 250, 251f
to femoral artery bypass, 248, 249f, 250, 251f, 252, 253f
in femoroperoneal bypass, 255f
posterior
in femoral anterior tibial bypass, 251f
to femoral bypass. See Femoral posterior tibial bypass.
in femoroperoneal bypass, 254, 255f
Tibial nerve
in femoral anterior tibial bypass, 251f
in femoropopliteal bypass, 228, 229f
Tibial vein, 245f, 251f
Tibialis anterior muscle, 250, 251f
Tibialis posterior muscle, 251f

U

Ultrasound, carotid, 3, 4
Ureter
in abdominal aortic aneurysm repair, 61f
in aortofemoral bypass, 198, 199f, 269f
in aortorenal bypass, 148, 149f, 155f

V

Vagus nerve
in carotid endarterectomy, 7f
injury to, 5
in innominate endarterectomy, 53f
in subclavian artery revascularization, 40, 41f
in vertebral artery revascularization, 47f
Valvulotome, 140, 141f, 242, 243f
Vein graft thrombosis, 278, 279f